The
Natu
PHARM

TNP.com

Inside—Find the Answers to These Questions and More

☑ Will taking calcium supplements help PMS symptoms? (See page 36.)

☑ Does creatine really improve sports performance? (See page 64.)

☑ Does glucosamine help relieve osteoarthritis? (See page 93.)

☑ Are high doses of beta-carotene supplements good for you? (See page 20.)

☑ Can chromium help weight loss? (See page 49.)

☑ What is SAMe, and can it help depression and osteoarthritis? (See page 192.)

☑ What is ipriflavone and can it help prevent osteoporosis? (See page 113.)

☑ Can phosphatidylserine improve mental function? (See page 173.)

☑ Will vitamin B₆ reduce the risk of heart disease? (See page 232.)

☑ Can zinc reduce cold symptoms? (See page 267.)

THE NATURAL PHARMACIST™ Library

Natural Health Bible,
Revised and Expanded 2nd Edition

Drug-Herb-Vitamin Interactions Bible

Illnesses and Their Natural Remedies

Herbs

Vitamins and Supplements

Migraines

Heart Disease Prevention

Anxiety

Arthritis

Colds and Flus

Diabetes

Cholesterol

Memory

Menopause

PMS

Reducing Cancer Risk

BPH (Prostate Enlargement)

Depression

Osteoporosis

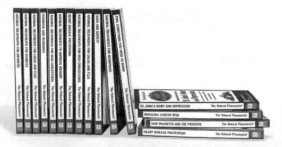

Visit us online at www.TNP.com

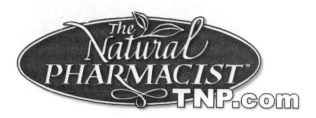

Your Complete Guide to
Vitamins
and Supplements

Angelo De Palma, Ph.D

Series Editors
Steven Bratman, M.D.
David Kroll, Ph.D.

A DIVISION OF PRIMA PUBLISHING
3000 Lava Ridge Court • Roseville, California 95661
(800) 632-8676 • www.primahealth.com

Published in association with TNP.com

Warning—Disclaimer
This book is not intended to provide medical advice and is sold with the understanding that the publisher and the author are not liable for the misconception or misuse of information provided. The author and Prima Publishing shall have neither liability nor responsibility to any person or entity with respect to any loss, damage, or injury caused or alleged to be caused directly or indirectly by the information contained in this book or the use of any products mentioned. Readers should not use any of the products discussed in this book without the advice of a medical professional.

TNP.COM, THE NATURAL PHARMACIST.COM, THE NATURAL PHARMACIST, and associated logo are trademarks of Prima Communications, Inc. The Prima Health logo is a registered trademark of Prima Communications, Inc., registered with the United States Patent and Trademark Office.

The Food and Drug Administration has not approved the use of any of the natural treatments discussed in this book. This book, and the information contained herein, has not been approved by the Food and Drug Administration.

All products mentioned in this book are trademarks of their respective companies.

Library of Congress Cataloging-in-Publication Data on file
ISBN 0-7615-1672-7

01 02 HH 10 9 8 7 6 5
Printed in the United States of America

How to Order
Single copies may be ordered from Prima Publishing, 3000 Lava Ridge Court, Roseville, CA 95661; telephone (800) 632-8676 ext. 4444. Quantity discounts are also available. On your letterhead, include information concerning the intended use of the books and the number of books you wish to purchase.

Visit us online at www.TNP.com and www.primahealth.com

Contents

What Makes This Book Different?

The interest in natural medicine has never been greater. According to the National Association of Chain Drug Stores, 65 million Americans are using natural supplements, and the number is growing! Yet it is hard for the consumer to find trustworthy sources for balanced information about this emerging field. Why? Frankly, natural medicine has had a checkered history. From snake oil potions sold at the turn of the century to those books, magazines, and product catalogs that hype miracle cures today, this is a field where exaggerated claims have been the norm. Proponents of natural medicine have tended to abuse science, treating it more as a marketing tool than a means of discovering the truth.

But there is truth to be found. Studies of vitamins, minerals, and other food supplements have been with us since these nutritional substances were first discovered, and the level and quality of this science has grown dramatically in the last 20 years. Herbal medicine has been neglected in the United States, but in Europe, this, the oldest of all healing arts, has been the subject of tremendous and ongoing scientific interest.

At present, for a number of herbs and supplements, it is possible to give reasonably scientific answers to the questions: How well does this work? How safe is it? What types of conditions is it best used for?

THE NATURAL PHARMACIST series is designed to cut through the hype and tell you what we know and what we don't know about popular natural treatments. These books are more conservative than any others available, more honest about the weaknesses of natural approaches, more fair in their comparisons of natural and conventional treatments. You won't find any miracle cures here, but you will discover useful options that can help you become healthier.

Why Choose Natural Treatments?

Although the science behind natural medicine continues to grow, this is still a much less scientifically validated field than conventional medicine. You might ask, "Why should I resort to an herb that is only partly proven, when I could take a drug with solid science behind it?" There are at least three good reasons to consider natural alternatives.

First, some herbs and supplements offer benefits that are not matched by any conventional drug. Vitamin E is a good example. It appears to help prevent prostate cancer, a benefit that no standard medication can claim.

Another example is the herb milk thistle. Studies strongly suggest that this herb can protect the liver from injury. There is no pill or tablet your doctor can prescribe to do the same.

Even if the science behind some of these treatments is less than perfect, when the risks are low and the possible benefit high, a treatment may be worth trying. It is a little-known fact that for many conventional treatments the science is less than perfect as well, and physicians must balance uncertain benefits against incompletely understood risks.

A second reason to consider natural therapies is that some may offer benefits comparable to those of drugs with fewer side effects. The herb St. John's wort is a good example. Reasonably strong scientific evidence suggests that this herb is an effective treatment for mild to moderate depression, while producing fewer side effects on average than conventional medications. Saw palmetto for benign enlargement of the prostate, ginkgo for relieving symptoms and perhaps slowing the progression of Alzheimer's disease, and glucosamine for osteoarthritis are other examples. This is not to say that herbs and supplements are completely harmless—they're not—but for most the level of risk is quite low.

Finally, there is a philosophical point to consider. For many people, it "feels" better to use a treatment that comes from nature instead of from a laboratory. Just as you might rather wear all-cotton clothing than polyester, or look at a mountain landscape rather than the skyscrapers of a downtown city, natural treatments may simply feel more compatible with your view of life. We can quibble endlessly about just what "natural" means and whether a certain treatment is "actually" natural or not, but such arguments are beside the point. The difference is in the feeling, and feelings matter. In fact, having a good feeling about taking an herb may lead you to use it more consistently than you would a prescription drug.

Of course, at times synthetic drugs may be necessary and even lifesaving. But on many other occasions it may be quite reasonable to turn to an herb or supplement instead of a drug.

To make good decisions you need good information. Unfortunately, while hundreds of books on alternative medicine are published every year, many are highly misleading. The phrase "studies prove" is often used when the studies in question are so small or so badly conducted that they prove nothing at all. You may even find that the "data" from other books come from studies with petri dishes and not real people!

You can't even assume that books written by well-known authors are scientifically sound. Many of these authors rely on secondary writers, leading to a game of "telephone," where misconceptions are passed around from book to book. And there's a strong tendency to exaggerate the power of natural remedies, whitewashing them with selective reporting.

THE NATURAL PHARMACIST series gives you the balanced information you need to make informed decisions about your health needs. Setting a new, high standard of accuracy and objectivity, these books take a realistic look at the herbs and supplements you read about in the news. You will encounter both favorable and unfavorable studies in these pages and will learn about both the benefits and the risks of natural treatments.

THE NATURAL PHARMACIST series is the source you can trust.

Steven Bratman, M.D.
David Kroll, Ph.D.

Introduction

Do vitamins and other nutritional supplements really work? Is there any science behind them? Are you protecting your future or wasting your money when you buy them?

Certainly, not all the claims you read about vitamins and supplements are true. However, there is actually a great deal of science behind the use of food supplements, much more research, in fact, than there is for herbs. This book will explain what we know and don't know about these popular and, in many cases, controversial treatments. It will tell you how to use them safely, economically, and to the best effect.

A Brief History of Dietary Supplements

The story of vitamins and food supplements goes back at least to 1748, when scurvy was a disastrous problem in the British navy. Surgeon's mate James Lind of the HMS *Salisbury* recruited 12 crew members with advanced scurvy and divided them into six groups, each of which received a different remedy for 6 days. When the crew members given citrus fruit showed dramatic recovery, he knew he was on to something important.

However, it wasn't until 1923 that ascorbic acid (vitamin C) was identified as the active "antiscurvy" ingredient in citrus fruit. Around the same time, many other essential nutrients were also discovered, eventually making up the vitamins and minerals now known to sustain life.

All together, these are known as *micronutrients,* meaning that you don't need very much of them in your diet to survive, compared with proteins, starches, and fats. Just grams or in some cases micrograms are enough.

When the essential micronutrients were first discovered, they were the province of conventional physicians, not advocates of natural medicine. Indeed, early writers in alternative medicine heavily criticized the use of vitamins. As the herbalist Jethro Kloss said in the introduction to his 1939 classic *Back to Eden* (Public Domain edition),[1] "Recently a Chicago firm advertised very extensively some little tablets claiming that they contained all the elements needed by the body, and were prepared by scientifically combining foods . . . [but] the most learned scientists who ever lived on this earth cannot separate natural foods and then combine them in a better manner than nature herself has prepared them."

However, the tide gradually turned in the 1950s and 1960s when Adelle Davis, and later Linus Pauling, began to publicize the benefits of vitamins and other nutritional substances. Soon, these became the mainstay of alternative medicine; today, along with herbs, dietary supplements compose most of the multibillion-dollar alternative health industry.

In recent decades, conventional medicine has once more begun to take an interest in the therapeutic use of these treatments. Research into their possible benefits has expanded dramatically, and major medical journals regularly run articles on using "drugs" such as vitamin E or selenium to prevent cancer.

Of course, vitamins aren't drugs in the ordinary sense. But there is an important issue to consider here: the distinction between nutritional and high-dose use of a supplement.

Nutritional Uses of Supplements

There is no doubt that we need to get a certain minimum of each essential nutrient to be healthy. Just as you can't run a car without gasoline, brake fluid, oil, transmission fluid, and antifreeze, you can't keep your body healthy without enough vitamins and minerals. And if you don't get enough of these nutrients through your diet, you need to get them some other way. Food supplements can be great insurance against the pitfalls of an inadequate diet.

When you take just enough of a nutrient to make sure you satisfy your needs, you can fairly say that you are taking a nutritional treatment or using nutritional supplementation. (The other way is to take very high dosages for a specific therapeutic effect, as described in the next section.) Supplements with real evidence that they may help prevent or treat disease when used at nutritional doses include vitamin B_6 and folic acid for prevention of heart disease, calcium for PMS symptoms, calcium plus vitamin D for osteoporosis, zinc and selenium for prevention of colds, gamma-linolenic acid (GLA) for diabetic neuropathy, fish oil (a source of essential fatty acids) for reducing symptoms of rheumatoid arthritis, and selenium for prevention of cancer.

But how much do you really need? It turns out that identifying necessary nutrients and determining the precise amount you really need is not an easy and straightforward task. Exact needs vary from person to person and even situation to situation, and although it is easy to observe the effects of severe deficiencies (such as scurvy), minor deficiencies are hard to measure. Thus, there is actually a lot of guesswork that goes into the recommendations for how much of a given nutrient you should take daily.

For some nutrients, such as chromium, the exact daily need is not known with any degree of certainty. In other cases, it may be that one dose sustains health whereas another improves it. Finally, many nutrients may not be absolutely necessary but may be helpful nonetheless when provided.

Various recommendations have been issued by governmental organizations at different times. In the United States, the most important include the Recommended Dietary Allowance (RDA), the Recommended Daily Value (RDV), the Dietary Reference Intake (DRI), the Estimated Average Requirements (EAR), and the Estimated Safe and Adequate Daily Dietary Intake (ESADDI). In Canada, the prevailing standard is the Recommended Nutrient Intake (RNI). Other standards have been set by the Food and Agricultural Organization and the World Health Organization of the United Nations, as well as by other individual countries.

In general, the recommendations of various governing bodies differ, by a little or a lot, depending on the nutrient. This book focuses on the U.S. RDA when one is available; otherwise it uses the ESADDI.

Because taking nutritional supplements is like an insurance policy, some people recommend taking more than you strictly need to make sure you get enough. This strategy makes sense for nutrients that don't easily become toxic; if you happen to get too much, it's a waste of money but no other problem. However, for potentially toxic vitamins and minerals (such as vitamins A and D, selenium, and zinc), caution is necessary. Also, dietary supplements are not cost-free. If you don't need to take 10 pills a day, maybe you don't want to. Under each supplement described in this book, we will discuss what is known about how much you need for nutritional purposes (see the heading Requirements/Sources) and point out the upper limits of safety.

Certain nutrients are commonly deficient in our diets, most prominently vitamin B_6, vitamin C, vitamin E, folate, magnesium, zinc, essential fatty acids, and calcium. Provided you take the right dosage, there is little to be lost and much to be gained by taking extra amounts of these supplements. In general, a good multivitamin and mineral tablet should contain enough of everything you need, but the last two in the list, essential fatty acids and calcium, need to be taken separately.

High Dosages of Supplements

Besides taking vitamins and minerals to supply nutrient needs, there is another very popular way to use them. Sometimes known as "megadose" treatment or "orthomolecular medicine," this approach involves taking amounts considerably beyond any reasonable nutritional need. In this book, these are described as "therapeutic dosages" and they are listed under a heading separate from that for requirements.

For example, the estimated dietary requirement of vitamin E is about 10 to 15 IU (international units) daily. But when used as an antioxidant supplement to prevent heart disease and prostate cancer, the typical recommended dosage is 400 to 800 IU daily—25 to 80 times higher than nutritional needs. There is simply no way you could ever get this much from food.

When you take megadoses of a vitamin, you are using it almost as a drug. It may act somewhat similarly to the way it works when taken at nutritional doses, or it may function entirely differently when present in such high concentrations. Even though vitamin E is a nutritional substance, this is not a nutritional treatment, properly speaking. It is a *therapeutic* use of vitamin E; in technical terms, a "supraphysiological" use (above normal bodily function).

It's hard to get too worried about the safety of supplements when taken at or near your nutritional needs. However, when they are used in gigantic doses, it is always possible that new health risks are created. In this book, we carefully distinguish between nutritional and high-dose use of all supplements described.

Examples of high-dose supplements with good research evidence behind them include vitamin E for prevention of cancer, vitamin C as well as zinc for reducing the severity and duration of colds, niacin for high cholesterol, magnesium for migraine headache prevention, and chromium for improving blood sugar control in people with diabetes.

Are All Dietary Supplements Nutrients?

The legal classification of dietary supplement is a bit vague. Besides essential nutrients, it includes other substances that are found in foods but may not be necessary in the diet, as well as substances related to those found in foods. For example, the sleep-inducing hormone melatonin is by no stretch of the imagination a nutritional substance, but because it is found in very low concentrations in bananas, it is legally marketed as a dietary supplement. Similarly, the synthetic substance ipriflavone (used for osteoporosis) is available as a dietary supplement because it is chemically related to a natural substance found in soybeans.

In some cases, the dietary supplement designation is simply a marketing technique that manufacturers use to avoid the expense of seeking drug approval. In others, the supplement is thought to work in at least a seminutritional way. For example, flavonoids, found in fruits and vegetables, are not essential nutrients, but the body may still use them when they are available and thereby receive health benefits. Another example is the supplement glucosamine, which is a substance found in cartilage. Although glucosamine is not an essential nutrient, it appears that supplemental glucosamine can help the body repair cartilage, thus reducing symptoms of arthritis.

In this book, we distinguish between true nutrients, seminutrients, and substances that are sold as nutrients but really aren't nutritional at all. Food supplements that aren't true nutrients but have relatively good evidence for their effectiveness include glucosamine and chondroitin for osteoarthritis, coenzyme Q_{10} for various forms of heart disease, oligomeric proanthocyanidins (OPCs) for varicose veins, soy for lowering cholesterol, lipoic acid for diabetic neuropathy, ipriflavone for osteoporosis, and phosphatidylserine for mental impairment.

How Do We Know If a Treatment Really Works?

The answer to this important question is much more complicated than it sounds. One might think "you just try it and see," but the reality is much more complex. If a treatment suddenly and dramatically cures a condition that is otherwise almost always fatal (such as penicillin for pneumonia), you really can discover its effectiveness just by paying attention. But most other cases are more difficult to pin down.

Suppose, for example, that you take vitamin C at the beginning of a cold and get better in 4 days. Was it the vitamin that helped? Would it have been a mild cold anyway? Or did you just convince yourself that you got better faster?

To make matters even more complex, the power of suggestion really can cure illnesses. In some studies, phony treatment (placebo) has significantly relieved symptoms in up to 70% of participants;[2] some trials using placebo have produced good results that are maintained for up to 18 months.[3]

This simply does not happen with cars, for example. If you turn a wrench and the engine runs better, you can be fairly certain it was your work and not the power of suggestion that caused the improvement. But if you try a supplement or a drug and notice an improvement in your symptoms, you can't be so sure that it was specifically the treatment that made the difference. This makes discovering effective treatments for diseases a surprisingly tricky process.

Over the last century medical science developed a way to get around the placebo effect: the *double-blind placebo-controlled study.* If you consider the subject carefully, you will realize that only this type of study can really prove that a treatment works.

In double-blind placebo-controlled studies, one group of study subjects receives the "real thing"—the active ingredient being tested. The other half receives a placebo designed to appear, as much as possible, like the real drug or supplement.

When scientists examine and report the results after the study is completed, they don't simply look at the improvement from the real drug or supplement. Saying "Those who took glucosamine experienced an average 50% reduction in arthritis symptoms" doesn't really mean much. Of course they improved: Because of the power of suggestion, they would definitely improve, no matter what.

Instead, researchers compare the results in the two groups. They report something like, "The glucosamine group experienced a 50% reduction in symptoms, compared with only a 30% reduction in the placebo group (also called the 'control' group)." It is the *difference* between the treatment group and the placebo group that shows whether a treatment is effective.

It is very important that neither the patient nor the doctor performing the study knows who is taking the drug or supplement and who is taking the placebo. This way, the power of suggestion doesn't cause participants to feel better (or worse); also, the doctor evaluating the participants is not biased in his or her assessment by knowing whether a given person is taking the real treatment or placebo. (Doctors can also subtly convey confidence or lack of it if they know who is receiving real treatment and who is not.)

If a study isn't double-blind, it is called an *open study,* and you have to take the results with a grain of salt. If only the participants are kept in the dark, but the doctors know which group is which, the study is called *single-blind.*

There is one more issue to keep in mind. Studies have to be reasonably large to prove much. Treatments that produce a relatively mild effect at best, such as vitamin C for reducing cold symptoms, need to include at least 100 people to make a good case, and 300 participants would be even better. Dramatically effective treatments can prove themselves in somewhat smaller trials. However, research involving 20 or fewer people generally doesn't prove anything at all. If you flip a coin 20 times, chances are pretty good that the number of heads and tails won't come out even, but this doesn't "prove" that the coin is biased.

Statisticians can analyze the results of a study to see whether the results really indicate anything. This analysis is called a *test for statistical significance.* If a study seems to show a benefit, but the results aren't statistically significant, you can't take the study to prove anything at all. In this book, unless stated otherwise, all results mentioned were found to be statistically significant.

Observational Versus Intervention Trials

For some diseases that occur relatively rarely, such as cancer, you need to involve many thousands of people to know if a treatment is exerting a useful preventive effect. The simplest way to look for such a benefit is to conduct what are called *observational studies.* However, they have many pitfalls.

Observational studies follow large groups of people for years and keep track of a great deal of information about them, including diet. Researchers then examine the data closely and try to identify which dietary factors are associated with better health and longer life.

However, the results can be misleading. For example, if an observational study finds that people who take vitamin supplements live longer, it is not necessarily the vitamins that deserve the credit. Vitamin users also tend to exercise more and to eat more healthful foods, habits that may play a more important role than the vitamins. It is hard to tell which factor is the most important. Researchers try to look closely at the data and eliminate such factors, but it can be very tricky to do so properly.

A more reliable kind of study is the *intervention trial*. In these studies, some people are given a certain vitamin and then compared with others who are given a placebo (a double-blind placebo-controlled trial is the best type of intervention trial). The results of intervention trials are far more conclusive than those of observational studies. Unfortunately, they are very expensive to perform when you need to enroll thousands of people. Relatively few have been completed.

Other Types of Studies

There are many other types of studies. Some don't prove much at all. Others have some meaning, but are not completely reliable.

An example of a study that proves little is the famous *in vitro*, or test-tube, study. Magazines never seem to tire of reporting old studies that found garlic capable of killing bacteria in test tubes. The obvious, but incorrect, conclusion is that when you eat garlic, it acts as an antibiotic. However, if you pour vinegar, orange juice, or bleach in a test tube, any one of these will also kill bacteria. These liquids don't work the same way when you drink them! Test-tube studies do not account for the fact that a substance given orally must be absorbed into the bloodstream, survive processing by the liver, and still manage to be effective when diluted by the fluids of the body. It's a long leap from a test tube to a real treatment.

In vitro studies are really only spurs to further research. They don't prove that a treatment is effective in real life.

There are many other examples of potentially misleading research. Studies that use injections instead of oral dosing can't be fully trusted because an injected substance doesn't have to run the gauntlet of the digestive tract. Evidence from animal studies can be very helpful, but because animals may process nutrients differently than we do, they can't be taken as completely reliable.

Perhaps the least reliable study relies on deficiencies as evidence that a supplement will work. The logic behind such claims goes like this: "People with diabetes have lower levels of XYZ nutrient in their blood; therefore, supplying more XYZ will improve diabetes." However, people with diabetes may be deficient in a particular nutrient because foods containing that nutrient are not part of their diet, or because diabetes affects their taste for that food and makes it unpalatable, or because *diabetes causes the deficiency*—not the other way around.

Finally, many basic scientific investigations show *how* a supplement might work but not that it *does* work. For example, zinc is essential for the proper function of the immune system, but this does not prove that taking extra zinc will strengthen your immunity. The gold standard is double-blind research, and in the following pages we will showcase those studies above all.

How Much Scientific Evidence Exists for Supplements?

Performing double-blind placebo-controlled studies is expensive. The top drug companies spend tens—even hundreds—of millions of dollars studying just one drug. Unless a company sees a good chance of recovering these costs, it will not even begin clinical studies. In addition, drug companies always take out one or more patents on a drug very early in its development. If the drug is eventually approved, the patent grants the company, for a set period of time, exclusive rights to make and sell the drug.

Unfortunately most vitamins and nutritional supplements cannot be patented because they were discovered decades ago. Without an exclusive right to a supplement, there is little chance any one company can recoup the millions required to conduct clinical trials on it. That is why quality clinical evidence is scarcer for most supplements than for medications.

As a reward for their investments in time and money, drug companies are allowed another benefit: They are permitted by law to make specific medical claims regarding their products—for example, "Lovastatin lowers cholesterol." Because most supplement companies have not tested their products according to U.S. Food and Drug Administration regulations, they generally cannot make such claims. They are limited to such vague statements as "Promotes healthy cholesterol."

Nonetheless, a great deal of good scientific investigation into the uses of vitamins and other food supplements has been done. Much of the funding has come from governmental sources looking for ways to improve public health.

This book will describe the latest research evidence for vitamins and other food supplements. When the evidence is strong, we will say so. When all the available research is still preliminary, we will say so as well. Treatments that are simply rumored to work but have little to no evidence behind them will still be listed and described honestly in case you wish to try them (they may still work—we just don't know for sure yet). And sometimes there is actually evidence that a popular treatment does not work, as you will be able to clearly see. The goal is to give you a sense of how much confidence you can place in a treatment you may consider trying.

A Word About Safety

Although a drug has to undergo extensive safety testing before it can be marketed, with a dietary supplement the situation is reversed: It cannot be removed from the shelves until proven dangerous. Fortunately, most commonly used supplements have a fairly high margin of safety.

This doesn't mean that they are all absolutely safe, however. The most common issues include safety in young children, pregnant or nursing women, individuals with severe illnesses, and those taking certain medications while also using supplements. Also, very high-dose supplementation and extensive long-term use of supplements may conceivably present certain risks. This book will tell you whatever is known or, in some cases, hypothesized about the safety of each supplement described.

The Limitations of This Book

Remember that no book can substitute for individualized medical care from a physician. Every person is different and has specific health needs only a doctor can assess. Furthermore, in many cases it is possible to use combinations of treatments—both natural and pharmaceutical—in sophisticated ways that cannot be described in a book of this type. The information contained in the following text should be regarded as an introduction, a suggestion for where to start.

5-HTP (5-HYDROXYTRYPTOPHAN)

Principal Proposed Uses
Depression, Migraine Headaches
Other Proposed Uses
Obesity (Weight Loss), Fibromyalgia, Anxiety, Insomnia

Many antidepressant drugs work, at least in part, by raising serotonin levels. The supplement 5-hydroxytryptophan (5-HTP) has been tried in cases of depression for a similar reason: the body uses 5-HTP to make serotonin, so providing the body with 5-HTP might therefore raise serotonin levels.

As a supplement, 5-HTP has also been proposed for all the same uses as other antidepressants, including aiding weight loss, preventing migraine headaches, decreasing the discomfort of fibromyalgia, improving sleep quality, and reducing anxiety.

Sources

5-HTP is not found in foods to any appreciable extent. For use as a supplement, it is manufactured from the seeds of an African plant *(Griffonia simplicifolia)*.

Therapeutic Dosages

A typical dosage of 5-HTP is 100 to 200 mg 3 times daily. Once 5-HTP starts to work, it may be possible to reduce the dosage significantly and still maintain good results.

Therapeutic Uses

The primary use of 5-HTP is for depression. Several small, short-term studies have found that it may be as effective as standard antidepressant drugs.[1,2] Since standard antidepressants are also used for insomnia and anxiety, 5-HTP has also been suggested as a treatment for those conditions, although there is as yet no direct evidence that it works.

Some, but not all, studies suggest that regular use of 5-HTP may help reduce the frequency and severity of migraine headaches.[3-8] Additionally, preliminary evidence suggests that 5-HTP can reduce symptoms of fibromyalgia[9] and perhaps help you lose weight.[10,11,12]

What Is the Scientific Evidence for 5-HTP?

Depression

Several small studies have compared 5-HTP to standard antidepressants.[13] The best one was a recent 6-week study of 63 people given either 5-HTP (100 mg 3 times daily) or an antidepressant in the Prozac family (fluvoxamine, 50 mg 3 times daily).[14] Researchers found equal benefit between the supplement and the drug. Actually, 5-HTP worked a little better at reducing depressed mood, anxiety, physical symptoms, and insomnia, but the differences were not statistically significant. There was no question that 5-HTP caused fewer and less severe side effects. The only real complaint with 5-HTP was occasional mild digestive distress, which is found with virtually all medications.

Migraine Headaches

A number of drugs are used to prevent migraine headaches, including antidepressants in the Prozac family. Although we don't know for sure, many of them appear to work by either changing serotonin levels or producing serotonin-like effects in the body. There is some evidence that 5-HTP may help prevent migraines too.

In a 6-month trial of 124 people, 5-HTP proved equally effective as the standard drug methysergide.[15] The most dramatic benefits seen were reductions in the intensity and duration of migraines. Since methysergide has been proven better than placebo for migraine headaches in earlier studies, the study results provide meaningful, although not airtight, evidence that 5-HTP is also effective.

Similarly good results were seen in another comparative study, using a different medication.[16]

However, in one study, 5-HTP was less effective than the drug propranolol.[17] Also, in a study involving children, 5-HTP failed to demonstrate benefit.[18] Other studies that are sometimes quoted as evidence that 5-HTP is effective for migraines actually enrolled adults or children with many different types of headaches (including migraines).[19,20,21]

Putting all this evidence together, it appears likely that 5-HTP can help people with frequent migraine headaches, but further research needs to be done. In particular, we need a large double-blind study that compares 5-HTP against placebo over a period of several months.

Obesity (Weight Loss)

The drug fenfluramine was one member of the now infamous phen-fen treatment for weight loss. Although very successful, fenfluramine was later associated with damage to the valves of the heart, and was removed from the market. Because fenfluramine raises serotonin levels, it seems reasonable to believe that other substances that affect serotonin might also be useful for weight reduction.

Three, small, placebo-controlled double-blind clinical trials have examined whether 5-HTP can help you lose weight. The first study found that 5-HTP (80 mg daily) could reduce caloric intake despite the fact that the 19 participants made no conscious effort to eat less.[22] The second study, which used a much higher dosage (900 mg daily) in 20 overweight women, found that treatment helped the participants stick to their diets.[23] The result was improved weight loss.

A third study that enrolled 20 obese women confirmed the results of the second, with slightly better results: After 12 weeks the average weight loss in the 5-HTP group was 10.3 pounds versus just 2.28 pounds in the placebo group.[24] These impressive results deserve more study.

(For another approach to weight loss, specifically reducing fat, see the chapter on chromium.)

Fibromyalgia

Antidepressants are the primary conventional treatment for fibromyalgia, a little-understood disease characterized by aching, tender muscles, fatigue, and disturbed sleep. One study suggests that 5-HTP may be helpful as well. In this double-blind trial, 50 subjects with fibromyalgia were given either 100 mg of 5-HTP or placebo 3 times daily for a month.[25] Those receiving 5-HTP experienced significant improvements in all symptom categories, including pain, stiffness, sleep patterns, anxiety, and fatigue.

(For another approach to fibromyalgia, see the chapter on SAMe.)

Safety Issues

No significant adverse effects have been reported in clinical trials of 5-HTP. Side effects appear to be limited to occasional mild digestive distress and possible allergic reactions.

However, there is one potentially serious concern. In 1998, the U.S. Food and Drug Administration reported detecting a chemical compound known as "peak X" in some 5-HTP products. Peak X has a frightening history involving a supplement related to 5-HTP: tryptophan. Until about 10 years ago, tryptophan was widely used as a sleep aid. However, it was taken off the market when thousands of people using the supplement developed a disabling and sometimes fatal blood disorder. This same contaminant, peak X, was found to be associated with that disaster.

Since the body turns tryptophan into 5-HTP, the latter has been marketed as a safe replacement for the banned amino acid. Until recently, it was assumed that 5-HTP could not possibly present the same risk as tryptophan because it is manufactured completely differently. However, the recent discovery that the same substance exists in batches of 5-HTP is worrisome. At this time, there is no other information from the FDA regarding specific cautions on using 5-HTP, but you should pay close attention to reports that may follow up on this finding.

Safety in young children, pregnant or nursing women, and those with liver or kidney disease has not been established (although, in some studies children have been given 5-HTP without any apparent harmful effects).

⚠ Interactions You Should Know About

If you are taking prescription antidepressants, including **MAO inhibitors**, **SSRIs**, or **tricyclics:** Do not take 5-HTP in addition except on a physician's advice. There is a chance you might raise serotonin levels too high.

If you are taking the Parkinson's disease medication **carbidopa:** Taking 5-HTP at the same time might cause skin changes similar to those that develop in the disease scleroderma.[26,27,28]

ACIDOPHILUS AND OTHER PROBIOTICS

Supplement Forms/Alternate Names
B. bifidus, L. acidophilus, L. bulgaricus, L. reuteri, S. thermophilus, Other "Probiotic" Bacteria

Principal Proposed Uses
Vaginal Infections, Irritable Bowel Syndrome, "Traveler's Diarrhea," Viral Diarrhea (in Children), Antibiotic-Associated Diarrhea

Other Proposed Uses
Strengthening Immunity, High Cholesterol, Canker Sores, Crohn's Disease, Ulcerative Colitis, Colon Cancer Prevention, Milk Allergies, Yeast Hypersensitivity Syndrome

Acidophilus is a "friendly" strain of bacteria used to make yogurt and cheese. Although we are born without it, acidophilus soon establishes itself in our intestines and helps prevent intestinal infections. Acidophilus also flourishes in the vagina, where it protects women against yeast infections.

Acidophilus is one of several helpful strains of bacteria known collectively as *probiotics* (literally, "pro life," indicating that they are bacteria that help rather than harm). Others include *L. bulgaricus, S. thermophilus, L. reuteri,* and *B. bifidus*. Your digestive tract is like a rain forest ecosystem, with billions of bacteria and yeasts rather than trees, frogs, and leopards. Some of these internal inhabitants are more helpful to your body than others. Acidophilus and related probiotic bacteria not only help the digestive tract function, they also reduce the presence of less healthful organisms by competing with them for the limited space available.

Antibiotics can disturb the balance of your "inner rain forest" by killing friendly bacteria. When this happens, harmful bacteria and yeasts can move in and flourish. This is why women taking antibiotics sometimes develop vaginal infections.

Conversely, it appears that the regular use of probiotics can help prevent vaginal infections and generally improve the health of the gastrointestinal system. Whenever you take antibiotics, you should probably take probiotics as well, and continue them for some time after you are done with the course of treatment. There is also some reason to believe that regular use of probiotics can reduce your risk of developing infectious diarrhea while traveling through foreign countries, as well as help prevent childhood diarrhea.

Sources

Although we believe that they are helpful and perhaps even necessary for human health, we don't have a daily requirement for probiotic bacteria. They are living creatures, not chemicals, so they can sustain themselves in your body unless something comes along to damage them, such as antibiotics.

Cultured dairy products such as yogurt and kefir are good sources of acidophilus and other probiotic bacteria. Supplements are widely available in powder, liquid, capsule, or tablet form. Grocery stores and natural food stores both carry milk that contains live acidophilus.

Therapeutic Dosages

Dosages of acidophilus are expressed not in grams or milligrams, but in billions of organisms. A typical daily dose should supply about 3 to 5 billion live organisms. Because this is not a drug but a living organism that you are trying to transplant to your digestive tract, the precise dosage is not so important. But you should take it regularly. Each time you do, you reinforce the beneficial bacterial colonies in your body, which may gradually push out harmful bacteria and yeasts growing there.

The downside of using a living organism is that probiotics may die on the shelf. In fact, a study reported in 1990 found that most acidophilus capsules on the market contained no living acidophilus.[1] The container label should guarantee living acidophilus (or bulgaricus, and so on) at the time of purchase, not just at the time of manufacture. Another approach is to eat acidophilus-rich foods such as yogurt, where the bacteria are most likely still alive.

To treat or prevent vaginal infections, mix 2 tablespoons of yogurt or the contents of a couple of capsules of acidophilus with warm water and use as a douche.

Finally, in addition to increasing your intake of probiotics, you can take fructo-oligosaccharides, supplements that can promote thriving colonies of helpful bacteria in the digestive tract. (Fructo-oligosaccharides are carbohydrates found in fruit. *Fructo* means "fruit," and an *oligosaccharide* is a type of carbohydrate.) Taking this supplement is like putting manure in a garden; it is thought to foster a healthy environment for the bacteria you want to have inside you. The typical daily dose of fructo-oligosaccharides is between 2 and 8 g.

Therapeutic Uses

In a few small studies, acidophilus has been found to be effective against vaginal yeast infections as well as those caused by the *Gardnerella* bacteria.[2]

Some evidence also suggests that acidophilus and other probiotics may be helpful for treating irritable bowel syndrome as well as viral diarrhea in children; it may also help prevent traveler's diarrhea and diarrhea caused by antibiotics.[3–12]

Preliminary evidence suggests that regular use of probiotics may improve immunity.[13,14]

A very preliminary double-blind study suggests that acidophilus can slightly decrease cholesterol levels.[15]

Probiotic treatment has also been proposed as a treatment for canker sores, Crohn's disease, and ulcerative colitis, and as a preventative measure against colon cancer; but there is no solid evidence that it is effective.

There is some evidence that probiotics can help reduce symptoms of milk allergies when added to milk.[16]

Finally, probiotics may be helpful in a condition known as *yeast hypersensitivity syndrome* (also known as chronic candidiasis, chronic candida, systemic candidiasis, or just candida). Although this syndrome is not recognized by conventional medicine, some practitioners of alternative medicine believe that it is a common problem that leads to numerous symptoms, including fatigue, digestive problems, frequent sinus infections, muscle pain, and mental confusion. Yeast hypersensitivity syndrome is said to consist of a population explosion of the normally benign candida yeast that live in the vagina and elsewhere in the body, coupled with a type of allergic sensitivity to it. Probiotic supplements are widely recommended for this condition because they establish large, healthy populations of friendly bacteria that compete with the candida that is trying to take up residence.

What Is the Scientific Evidence for Acidophilus?

Vaginal Yeast Infections

A review of the many studies on the use of oral and topical acidophilus to prevent vaginal yeast infections concluded that the treatment was effective.[17]

Irritable Bowel Syndrome

People with irritable bowel syndrome (IBS) experience crampy digestive pain as well as alternating diarrhea and constipation and other symptoms. Although the cause of irritable bowel syndrome is not known, one possibility is a disturbance in healthy intestinal bacteria. Based on this theory, acidophilus has been tried as a treatment for IBS.

In a small double-blind study, 18 individuals with irritable bowel syndrome were given either placebo or a capsule containing 5 billion *L. acidophilus* organisms daily for 6 weeks.[18] Greater improvement was seen in the treated group than in the placebo group, but so many people dropped out of the study the results are difficult to evaluate.

Diarrhea

According to several studies, it appears that regular use of acidophilus and other probiotics can help prevent "traveler's diarrhea" (an illness caused by eating contaminated food, usually in developing countries).[19,20] One double-blind placebo-controlled study followed 820 individuals traveling to southern Turkey, and found that use of a probiotic called *Lactobacillus GG* significantly protected against intestinal infection.[21]

Probiotics may also help prevent or treat diarrhea in children. A double-blind study evaluated the possible benefits of the probiotic *L. reuteri* in 66 children with rotavirus diarrhea (rotavirus is a virus that can cause severe diarrhea in children).[22] The study found that treatment shortened the duration of symptoms, and the higher the dose, the better the effect.

Another double-blind placebo-controlled study found that *B. bifidum* and *S. thermophilus* can help protect against rotavirus infection in hospitalized infants.[23] A probiotic called *L. casei* may also help prevent diarrhea in children.[24]

Keep in mind that diarrhea in young children can be serious. If it persists for more than a day, you should take your child to a physician.

Probiotics may also help reduce antibiotic-related diarrhea.[25,26]

Immunity

A number of studies suggest that various probiotics can enhance immune function,[27] but there is only one double-blind placebo-controlled study on the subject. This 12-week trial evaluated 25 healthy elderly individuals, half of whom were given milk containing a particular strain of *Bifidobacterium lactis*, the others milk alone.[28] The results showed various changes in immune parameters which the researchers took as possibly indicating improved immune function.

Safety Issues

There are no known safety problems with the use of acidophilus or other probiotics. Occasionally, some people notice a temporary increase in digestive gas.

⚠ Interactions You Should Know About

If you are taking **antibiotics**, it may be beneficial to take probiotic supplements at the same time, and to continue them for a couple of weeks after you have finished the course of drug treatment. This will help restore the balance of natural bacteria in your digestive tract.

ANDROSTENEDIONE

Principal Proposed Uses
Athletic Performance

Androstenedione is a hormone produced naturally in the body by the adrenal glands, the ovaries (in women), and the testicles (in men). The body first manufactures DHEA, then turns DHEA into androstenedione, and finally transforms androstenedione into testosterone, the principal male sex hormone. Androstenedione is also transformed into estrogen.

Androstenedione is widely used by athletes who believe that it can build muscle and increase strength. However, there is no evidence that it works. U.S. baseball fans know that the all-time single-season home run champion, Mark McGwire, used androstenedione during his record-setting season. Whether it helped is anyone's guess. Hitting home runs is not only a matter of strength, but of timing and concentration as well. Nonetheless, if McGwire were playing in any other professional sport, or in the Olympics, he would have been suspended for using androstenedione.

Sources

Androstenedione is not an essential nutrient—your body manufactures it from scratch. It is found in meat and in some plants, but to get a therapeutic dosage, you will need to take supplements.

Therapeutic Dosages

The typical recommended dose of androstenedione is 100 mg 2 times daily with food.

Therapeutic Uses

Androstenedione is said to enhance athletic performance and strength by increasing testosterone production, thereby building muscle. However, the balance of evidence suggests that the supplement increases estrogen levels more than it increases testosterone levels, and that it doesn't enhance athletic performance. [1–4]

What Is the Scientific Evidence for Androstenedione?

In a 7-day, open study of 42 healthy men, 300 mg daily of androstenedione significantly increased testosterone levels.[5]

However, in an 8-week, double-blind placebo-controlled study of 20 healthy men undergoing weight training, 300 mg of androstenedione daily did not affect testosterone levels.[6]

A third trial also failed to find any change in testosterone levels among men given 200 mg of androstenedione daily.[7]

On balance, it does not appear that androstenedione increases testosterone. However, one fact was consistent in all these trials: androstenedione increased estrogen levels significantly. This change would not be expected to improve sports performance. Indeed, in the 8-week trial mentioned previously, no improvement in sports performance was seen.[8]

A 12-week, double-blind study of 40 trained male athletes given either DHEA or androstenedione at 100 mg daily also found no improvement in lean body mass or strength, or change in testosterone levels.[9]

Safety Issues

Androstenedione can cause hair loss on the head and growth of body hair.[10] There are also concerns that androstenedione, like related hormones, might increase the risk of liver cancer and heart disease. In addition, elevated estrogen levels could increase cancer risk in women.

Putting all this information together, we think it is fair to say that more research is needed before androstenedione can be recommended.

⚠ Interactions You Should Know About

If you are taking any **hormones** or **drugs that affect hormone levels**, it is possible that androstenedione might interfere.

AORTIC GLYCOSAMINOGLYCANS

Supplement Forms/Alternate Names
Aortic GAGs, Chondroitin Polysulphate, Chondroitin Sulfate A, CSA, Mesoglycan, Mucopolysaccharide

Principal Proposed Uses
Atherosclerosis, High Cholesterol, Varicose Veins, Hemorrhoids, Phlebitis

Aortic glycosaminoglycans (GAGs) are important substances found in many tissues in the body, including the joints and the lining of blood vessels. Chemically, aortic GAGs are related to the blood-thinning drug heparin and the supplement chondroitin (for more information, see the chapter on chondroitin). Unlike chondroitin, aortic GAGs are primarily used to treat diseases of blood vessels. Preliminary evidence suggests that aortic GAGs may be helpful for atherosclerosis, varicose veins, phlebitis, and hemorrhoids.

Sources

Aortic GAGs are not essential nutrients because the body usually manufactures them from scratch. For supplement purposes, aortic GAGs are commercially extracted from the aorta (the largest artery) of cows—hence the name. Substances very similar to aortic GAGs can be produced from cartilage, bone, or chondroitin sulfate, and are often used interchangeably.

Therapeutic Dosages

The usual dosage of aortic GAGs is 100 mg daily.

Therapeutic Uses

Hardening of the arteries due to atherosclerosis is the major cause of heart disease and strokes. High cholesterol, hypertension, cigarette smoking, and other factors damage the inner lining of blood vessels, causing a series of dangerous changes.

There is some evidence that aortic GAGs may slow the development of atherosclerosis, by lowering cholesterol levels, "thinning" the blood, or through other effects.[1,2,3]

They may also be useful for various other diseases of blood vessels, including varicose veins, hemorrhoids, and phlebitis.[4–7]

Warning: Do not self-treat phlebitis. It is a potentially deadly disease.

What Is the Scientific Evidence for Aortic Glycosaminoglycans?

Atherosclerosis

In a recent study, one group of men with early hardening of the coronary (heart) arteries was given 200 mg daily of aortic GAGs, while the other group received no treatment.[8] After 18 months, the layering of the vessel lining was 7.5 times greater in the untreated group than in the aortic GAG group, a significant difference. Additional preliminary evidence that aortic GAGs might help atherosclerosis comes from other studies in animals and people.[9,10] However, in the absence of properly designed double-blind trials, the results can't be taken as truly reliable.

We don't know how aortic GAGs might help atherosclerosis. There is some evidence that they can reduce cholesterol levels and also "thin" the blood.[11]

Vein Diseases

Several Italian studies suggest that aortic GAGs may be helpful in varicose veins, phlebitis, and hemorrhoids.[12–15] However, because the full text of these studies is not available in English, it is difficult to evaluate their merits.

Safety Issues

Aortic GAGs are essentially ground-up blood vessels from cows, so they are probably safe to take even in large quantities. The only concern that has been raised regards their ability to slightly decrease blood clotting (see Interactions You Should Know About). Maximum safe dosages for young children, pregnant or nursing women, or those with severe liver or kidney disease have not been determined.

⚠ Interactions You Should Know About

If you are taking drugs that powerfully decrease blood clotting, such as **Coumadin (warfarin)**, **heparin**, **Trental** (**pentoxifylline**), or even **aspirin**, do not use aortic GAGs except under physician supervision. Because aortic GAGs interfere slightly with blood clotting, there is a chance that the combination could cause bleeding problems.

ARGININE

Supplement Forms/Alternate Names
Arginine Hydrochloride, L-Arginine

Principal Proposed Uses
Colds (Prevention), Intermittent Claudication, Congestive Heart Failure, Male Infertility

Other Proposed Uses
Impotence

Arginine is an amino acid found in many foods, including dairy products, meat, poultry, and fish. It plays a role in several important mechanisms in the body, including cell division, the healing of wounds, the removal of ammonia from the body, immune function, and the secretion of important hormones.

The body also uses arginine to make nitric oxide, which relaxes the blood vessels. Based on this, arginine has been proposed as a treatment for various heart conditions, including congestive heart failure, and for impotence, which may be caused by limited blood flow. For reasons that are not at all clear, regular use of arginine may also be able to help reduce the frequency of colds.

Requirements/Sources

Normally, the body either gets enough arginine from food, or manufactures all it needs from other widely available nutrients. Certain stresses, such as severe burns, infections, and injuries, can deplete your body's supply of arginine.

Arginine is found in dairy products, meat, poultry, fish, nuts, and chocolate.

Therapeutic Dosages

A typical supplemental dosage of arginine is 2 to 3 g per day. For congestive heart failure, dosages as high as 30 g per day have been tried.

Warning: Do not try to self-treat congestive heart failure. If you have this condition, be sure to consult your physician before taking any supplements.

Therapeutic Uses

One preliminary double-blind study suggests that arginine supplementation might help prevent colds.[1]

Other preliminary studies suggest that arginine may relieve some of the symptoms of intermittent claudication[2] and congestive heart failure.[3,4] The supplement coenzyme Q_{10} (CoQ_{10}), however, has far better evidence as a treatment for the latter condition.

Preliminary evidence suggests that arginine may improve sperm function and thereby help treat male infertility, but not all studies have found benefit.[5–10]

Arginine has recently become popular as a male aphrodisiac and a cure for impotence, but there is little to no evidence that it works.

What Is the Scientific Evidence for Arginine?

Colds

A double-blind study involving 41 children concluded that arginine seemed to provide some protection against respiratory infections.[11] In this study, 20 children were given arginine and 20 received placebo for 60 days of the study. Of the children who received placebo, 15 developed minor respiratory infections (colds) during the 60 days of the study. By contrast, only 5 of the children taking arginine developed colds, a significant difference.

Intermittent Claudication

People with advanced hardening of the arteries, or athero-sclerosis, often have difficulty walking due to lack of blood flow to the legs, a condition known as intermittent claudication. Pain may develop after walking less than half a block. Food bars containing arginine have been found to improve walking distance. After 2 weeks of two food bars daily, study participants could walk 66% farther.[12]

Safety Issues

Arginine is an amino acid found naturally in our bodies and our food, and for this reason is believed to be quite safe. However, maximum safe dosages are not known for young children, pregnant or nursing women, or those with severe liver or kidney disease.

Keep in mind that the recommended dosage of arginine is so high that even low percentage levels of a contaminant might cause problems. Therefore, be sure to purchase a high-quality product.

⚠ Interactions You Should Know About

If you are taking **lysine** to treat herpes, arginine might counteract any potential benefit.

BCAAs

Supplement Forms/Alternate Names
Branched-Chain Amino Acids (Combined) or Leucine, Isoleucine, or Valine Separately

Principal Proposed Uses
Loss of Appetite (in Cancer Patients), Amyotrophic Lateral Sclerosis (ALS, Lou Gehrig's Disease)

Other Proposed Uses
Recovery From Surgery, Improving Athletic Performance, Muscular Dystrophy, Tardive Dyskinesia

Branched-chain amino acids (BCAAs) are naturally occurring molecules (leucine, isoleucine, and valine) that the body uses to build proteins. The term "branched chain" refers to the molecular structure of these particular amino acids. Muscles have a particularly high content of BCAAs.

For reasons that are not entirely clear, BCAA supplements may improve appetite in cancer patients and slow the progression of amyotrophic lateral sclerosis (ALS, or Lou Gehrig's disease, a terrible condition that leads to degeneration of nerves, atrophy of the muscles, and eventual death).

BCAAs have also been proposed as a supplement to boost athletic performance.

Requirements/Sources

Dietary protein usually provides all the BCAAs you need. However, physical stress and injury can increase your need for BCAAs to repair damage, so supplementation may be helpful.

BCAAs are present in all protein-containing foods, but the best sources are red meat and dairy products. Chicken, fish, and eggs are excellent sources as well. Whey protein and egg protein supplements are another way to ensure you're getting enough BCAAs. Supplements may contain all three BCAAs together or simply individual BCAAs.

Therapeutic Dosages

The typical dosage of BCAAs is 1 to 5 g daily.

Therapeutic Uses

Preliminary evidence suggests that BCAAs may improve appetite in cancer patients.[1] There is also some evidence that BCAA supplements may reduce symptoms of amyotrophic lateral sclerosis (ALS, or Lou Gehrig's disease).[2] Reports, but little real evidence, suggest that BCAAs may reduce muscle loss during recovery from surgery.

One very small open study (nine participants) suggests that BCAAs might possibly be helpful for tardive dyskinesia, a late-developing side effect of drugs used for psychosis.[3]

BCAAs have also been tried by athletes to build muscle; however, evidence suggests that they do not improve performance or enhance the muscle/fat ratio in the body.[4] BCAAs also do not appear to be helpful for muscular dystrophy.[5]

What Is the Scientific Evidence for BCAAs?

Appetite in Cancer Patients

A double-blind study tested BCAAs on 28 people with cancer who had lost their appetites due to either the disease itself or its treatment.[6] Appetite improved in 55% of those taking BCAAs (4.8 g daily) compared to only 16% of those who took placebo.

Amyotrophic Lateral Sclerosis (Lou Gehrig's Disease)

A small double-blind study suggested that BCAAs might help protect muscle strength in people with Lou Gehrig's disease.[7] Eighteen individuals were given either BCAAs (taken 4 times daily between meals) or placebo, and followed for 1 year. The results showed that people taking BCAAs declined much more slowly than those receiving placebo. In the placebo group, five of nine participants lost their ability to walk, two died, and another required a respirator. Only one of nine of those receiving BCAAs became unable to walk during the study period. This study is too small to give conclusive evidence, but it does suggest that BCAAs might be helpful for this disease.

Muscular Dystrophy

One double-blind placebo-controlled study found leucine ineffective at the dose of 0.2 g per kilogram body weight (15 g daily for a 75-kilogram woman) in 96 individuals with muscular dystrophy.[8] Over the course of 1 year, no differences were seen between the effects of leucine and placebo.

Safety Issues

BCAAs are believed to be safe; when taken in excess, they are simply converted into other amino acids. However, like other amino acids, BCAAs may interfere with medications for Parkinson's disease.

⚠ Interactions You Should Know About

If you are taking **medication for Parkinson's disease** (such as levodopa), BCAAs may reduce its effectiveness.

BETA-CAROTENE

Principal Proposed Uses
Heart Disease Prevention, Cataract Prevention, Macular Degeneration Prevention

Other Proposed Uses
Osteoarthritis, Easy Sunburning, AIDS, Alcoholism, Asthma, Depression, Epilepsy, Infertility, Headaches, Heartburn, Hypertension (High Blood Pressure), Parkinson's Disease, Psoriasis, Rheumatoid Arthritis, Schizophrenia

Probably Ineffective Uses
Cancer Prevention

Note: All the significant positive evidence for beta-carotene applies to food sources, not supplements.

Note: Beta-carotene and vitamin A are sometimes described as if they were the same thing. This is because the body converts beta-carotene into vitamin A. However, there are important differences between the two.

Beta-carotene belongs to a family of natural chemicals known as carotenes or carotenoids. Scientists have identified nearly 600 different carotenes (for information about other carotenes, see the chapters on lycopene and lutein). Widely found in plants, carotenes (along with another group of chemicals, the bioflavonoids) give color to fruits, vegetables, and other plants.

Beta-carotene is a particularly important carotene from a nutritional standpoint, because the body easily transforms it to vitamin A. While vitamin A supplements themselves can be toxic when taken to excess, if you take beta-carotene, your body will make only as much vitamin A as you need. This built-in safety feature makes beta-carotene the best way to get your vitamin A.

Beta-carotene is also often recommended for another reason: it is an antioxidant, like vitamin E and vitamin C. However, although there is a great deal of evidence that the carotenes found in food can provide a variety of health benefits (from reducing the risk of cancer to preventing heart disease), there is little to no evidence that high doses of purified beta-carotene supplements are good for you.

Requirements/Sources

Although beta-carotene is not an essential nutrient, vitamin A is. Three mg (5,000 IU) of beta-carotene supplies about 5,000 IU of vitamin A. (See the chapter on vitamin A for requirements based on age and sex.)

Dark green and orange-yellow vegetables are good sources of beta-carotene. These include carrots, sweet potatoes, squash, spinach, romaine lettuce, broccoli, apricots, and green peppers.

Therapeutic Dosages

We are not sure at the present time whether it is advisable to take dosages of beta-carotene much higher than the recommended allowance for nutritional purposes. It is probably much better to increase your intake of fresh fruits and veg etables.

Therapeutic Uses

It is difficult to recommend beta-carotene supplements for any use other than to supply nutritional levels of vitamin A.

Evidence suggests that mixed carotenes found in food can protect against cancer and heart disease.[1–7] However, supplements that contain only purified beta-carotene may actually be harmful for these conditions.[8–12]

Similarly, although mixed carotenes found in food seem to slow the progression of cataracts and help prevent macular degeneration, beta-carotene alone does not seem to work.[13–17]

Dietary beta-carotene may also slow down the progression of osteoarthritis, but we don't know whether beta-carotene supplements work for this purpose.[18]

Beta-carotene supplements may be helpful for people with extreme sensitivity to the sun, but the evidence is somewhat contradictory.[19–22] Finally, beta-carotene has been proposed as a treatment for AIDS, alcoholism, asthma, depression, epilepsy, headaches, heartburn, hypertension, male and female infertility, Parkinson's disease, psoriasis, rheumatoid arthritis, and schizophrenia, but there is little to no evidence that it works.

According to a double-blind placebo-controlled study of 141 women with cervical dysplasia (early cervical cancer), beta-carotene, taken at a dosage of 30 mg daily, does not help to reverse the dysplasia.[23]

What Is the Scientific Evidence for Beta-Carotene?

Cancer Prevention

The story of beta-carotene and cancer is full of contradictions. It starts in the early 1980s, when the cumulative results of many studies suggested that people who eat a lot of fruits and vegetables are significantly less likely to get cancer.[24,25] A close look at the data pointed to carotenes as the active ingredients in fruits and vegetables. It appeared that a high intake of dietary carotene could dramatically reduce the risk of lung cancer,[26] bladder cancer,[27] breast cancer,[28] esophageal cancer,[29] and stomach cancer.[30]

The next step was to give carotenes to people and see if it made a difference. Researchers used purified beta-carotene instead of mixed carotenes, because it is much more readily available. They studied people in high-risk groups, such as smokers, because it is easier to see results when you look at people who are more likely to develop cancer to begin with. However, the results were surprisingly unfavorable.

The anticancer bubble burst for beta-carotene in 1994 when the results of the Alpha-Tocopherol, Beta-Carotene

(ATBC) study came in.[31] These results showed that beta-carotene supplements did not prevent lung cancer, but actually increased the risk of getting it by 18%. This trial had followed 29,133 male smokers in Finland who took supplements of about 50 IU of vitamin E (alpha-tocopherol), 20 mg of beta-carotene, both, or placebo daily for 5 to 8 years. (In contrast, vitamin E was found to reduce the risk of cancer, especially prostate cancer. For more information, see the chapter on vitamin E.)

In January 1996, researchers monitoring the Beta-Carotene and Retinol Efficacy Trial (CARET) confirmed the prior bad news with more of their own: The beta-carotene group had 46% more cases of lung cancer deaths.[32] This study involved smokers, former smokers, and workers exposed to asbestos. Alarmed, the National Cancer Institute ended the $42 million CARET trial 21 months before it was planned to end.

At about the same time, the 12-year Physicians' Health Study of 22,000 male physicians was finding that 50 mg of beta-carotene taken every other day had no effect—good or bad—on the risk of cancer or heart disease. In this study, 11% of the participants were smokers and 39% were ex-smokers.[33] Interestingly, higher levels of carotene intake from diet were associated with lower levels of cancer.

What is the explanation for this apparent discrepancy? It could be that beta-carotene alone is not effective. The other carotenes found in fruits and vegetables may be more important for preventing cancer than beta-carotene. One researcher has suggested that taking beta-carotene supplements actually depletes the body of other beneficial carotenes.[34]

Heart Disease Prevention

The situation with beta-carotene and heart disease is rather similar to that of beta-carotene and cancer. Numerous studies suggest that carotenes as a whole can reduce the risk of heart disease.[35] However, isolated beta-carotene may not help prevent heart disease and could actually increase your risk.

The same double-blind intervention trial involving 29,133 Finnish male smokers (mentioned under the discussion of cancer and beta-carotene) found 11% more deaths from heart disease and 15 to 20% more strokes in those participants taking beta-carotene supplements.[36]

Similar poor results with beta-carotene were seen in another large double-blind study of smokers.[37] Beta-carotene supplementation was also found to increase the incidence of angina in smokers.[38]

The bottom line: as with cancer, the mixed carotenoids found in foods seem to be helpful for heart disease, but beta-carotene supplements do not.

Osteoarthritis
A high dietary intake of beta-carotene appears to slow the progression of osteoarthritis by as much as 70%, according to a study in which researchers followed 640 individuals over a period of 8 to 10 years.[39] However, again, we don't know if purified beta-carotene supplements work the same way as beta-carotene from food sources.[40]

Safety Issues
At recommended dosages, beta-carotene is very safe. The only side effects reported from beta-carotene overdose are diarrhea and a yellowish tinge to the hands and feet. These symptoms disappear once you stop taking beta-carotene or move to lower doses.

However, high-dose beta-carotene may slightly increase the risk of heart disease and cancer, especially in those who consume too much alcohol.[41] The solution: eat plenty of fresh fruits and vegetables, and get your beta-carotene that way.

BETAINE HYDROCHLORIDE

Principal Proposed Uses

There are no well-documented uses for betaine hydrochloride.

Other Proposed Uses

Digestive Aid, Anemia, Asthma, Atherosclerosis, Diarrhea, Excess Candida (Yeast), Food Allergies, Gallstones, Hay Fever, Inner Ear Infections, Rheumatoid Arthritis, Thyroid Conditions, Ulcers, Heartburn

Betaine hydrochloride is a source of hydrochloric acid, a naturally occurring chemical in the stomach that helps us digest food by breaking up fats and proteins. Stomach acid also aids in the absorption of nutrients through the walls of the intestines into the blood and protects the gastrointestinal tract from harmful bacteria.

A major branch of alternative medicine known as naturopathy has long held that low stomach acid is a widespread problem that interferes with digestion and the absorption of nutrients. Betaine hydrochloride is one of the most common recommendations for this condition (along with the more folksy apple cider vinegar).

Betaine is also sold by itself, without the hydrochloride molecule attached. In this form, it is called trimethylglycine (TMG). TMG is not acidic, but recent evidence suggests that it may provide certain health benefits of its own (for more information, see the chapter on TMG).

Sources

Betaine hydrochloride is not an essential nutrient, and no food sources exist.

Therapeutic Dosages

Betaine hydrochloride is typically taken in pill form at dosages ranging from 325 to 650 mg with each meal.

Therapeutic Uses

Based on theories about the importance of stomach acid, betaine has been recommended for a wide variety of problems, including anemia, asthma, atherosclerosis, diarrhea, excess candida yeast, food allergies, gallstones, hay fever and allergies, inner ear infections, rheumatoid arthritis, and thyroid conditions. When one sees such broadly encompassing uses, it is not surprising to find that there is as yet no real scientific research on its effectiveness for any of these conditions.

Many naturopathic physicians also believe that betaine hydrochloride can heal conditions such as ulcers and esophageal reflux (heartburn). This sounds paradoxical, since conventional treatment for those conditions involves reducing stomach acid, while betaine hydrochloride increases it. However, according to one theory, lack of stomach acid leads to incomplete digestion of proteins, and these proteins cause allergic reactions and other responses that lead to an increase in ulcer pain. Again, scientific evidence is lacking.

Safety Issues

Betaine hydrochloride should not be used by those with ulcers or esophageal reflux (heartburn) except on the advice of a physician. This supplement seldom causes any obvious side effects, but it has not been put through rigorous safety studies. In particular, safety for young children, pregnant or nursing women, or those with severe liver or kidney disease has not been established.

Biotin

Supplement Forms/Alternate Names
Biocytin (Brewer's Yeast–Biotin Complex)
Principal Proposed Uses
There are no well-documented uses for biotin.
Other Proposed Uses
Diabetes, Brittle Nails, "Cradle Cap" in Children

Biotin is a water-soluble B vitamin that plays an important role in metabolizing the energy we get from food. Biotin assists four essential enzymes that break down fats, carbohydrates, and proteins.

Very preliminary evidence suggests that biotin supplements may be helpful for people with diabetes.

Requirements/Sources

Although biotin is a necessary nutrient, we usually get enough from bacteria living in the digestive tract. Actual biotin deficiency is uncommon, unless you frequently eat large quantities of raw egg white. (Raw egg white contains a protein that blocks the absorption of biotin. Fortunately, cooked egg white does not present this problem.)

There is no recommended dietary allowance for biotin, but the Estimated Safe and Adequate Daily Dietary Intake is

- Infants under 6 months, 10 mcg
  6 to 12 months, 15 mcg
- Children 1 to 3 years, 20 mcg
  4 to 6 years, 25 mcg
  7 to 10 years, 30 mcg
- Adults (and children 11 years and older), 30 to 100 mcg

Good dietary sources of biotin include brewer's yeast, nutritional (torula) yeast, whole grains, nuts, egg yolks, sardines, legumes, liver, cauliflower, bananas, and mushrooms.

Therapeutic Dosages

For people with diabetes, the usual recommended dosage of biotin is 7,000 to 15,000 mcg daily.

For treating "cradle cap" (a scaly head rash often found in infants), the usual dosage of biotin is 6,000 mcg daily, *given to the nursing mother* (not the child). A lower dosage of 3,000 mcg daily is used to treat brittle fingernails and toenails.

Therapeutic Uses

There is little hard evidence for any of the proposed uses of biotin. Highly preliminary evidence suggests that supplemental biotin can help reduce blood sugar levels in people with either type 1 (childhood onset) or type 2 (adult onset) diabetes.[1,2] Biotin may also reduce the symptoms of diabetic neuropathy.[3] However, other supplements often recommended for diabetes have much better evidence behind them, such as chromium, lipoic acid, and GLA from evening primrose oil.

Even weaker evidence suggests that biotin supplements can promote healthy nails[4] and eliminate cradle cap.

Safety Issues

Biotin appears to be quite safe. However, maximum safe dosages for young children, pregnant or nursing women, or those with severe liver or kidney disease have not been established.

⚠ Interactions You Should Know About

If you are taking

- The antiseizure medications **carbamazepine** or **Mysoline (primidone):** Take biotin supplements at a different time of day.
- **Alcohol:** You may need extra biotin.

BORON

Supplement Forms/Alternate Names
Boron Chelate, Sodium Borate

Principal Proposed Uses
Osteoarthritis

Other Proposed Uses
Osteoporosis, Rheumatoid Arthritis

Plants need boron for proper health, but it's not known whether humans do. However, boron does seem to assist in the proper absorption of calcium, magnesium, and phosphorus from foods, and slows the loss of these minerals through urination. Very preliminary evidence suggests that boron may be helpful for arthritis and osteoporosis.

Sources

No dietary or nutritional requirement for boron has been established, and boron deficiency is not known to cause any disease. Good sources include leafy vegetables, raisins, prunes, nuts, non-citrus fruits, and grains. A typical American daily diet provides 1.5 to 3 mg of boron.

Therapeutic Dosages

When used as a treatment for arthritis or osteoporosis, boron is often recommended at a dosage of 3 mg per day, an amount similar to the average daily intake from food. However, food sources may be safer (see Safety Issues).

Therapeutic Uses

Although boron is often added to supplements intended for the treatment of osteoarthritis, the evidence that it helps is very weak.[1,2,3] Three other supplements—glucosamine, chondroitin, and SAMe—are much better researched treatments for osteoarthritis.

Boron has also been suggested as a treatment for osteoporosis.[4] (See the chapters on isoflavones, calcium, and vitamin D for more information on how to prevent or even reverse osteoporosis.)

Finally, boron is sometimes recommended as a treatment for rheumatoid arthritis, but there is no real evidence that it works.

What Is the Scientific Evidence for Boron?

Osteoarthritis

In areas of the world where people eat relatively high amounts of boron—between 3 and 10 mg per day—the incidence of osteoarthritis is below 10%. However, in regions where there is less boron in the diet—1 mg or less per day—the incidence of arthritis is higher.[5] This observation has given rise to the theory that boron supplements might be helpful for people who already have arthritis symptoms.

However, the only direct evidence that it works comes from one highly preliminary study.[6,7]

Osteoporosis

In one small study, 13 postmenopausal women were first fed a diet that provided 0.25 mg of boron for 119 days; then they were fed the same diet with a boron supplement of 3 mg daily for 48 days.[8] The results revealed that boron supplementation reduced the amount of calcium lost in the urine. This suggests (but certainly doesn't prove) that boron can help prevent osteoporosis. A more recent study failed to support this finding.[9]

Safety Issues

Since the therapeutic dosage of boron is about the same as the amount you can get from food, it is probably fairly safe. Unpleasant side effects, including nausea and vomiting, are only reported at about 50 times the highest recommended dose.

One potential concern with boron regards its effect on hormones. In at least two small studies, boron was found to increase the body's own estrogen levels, especially in women on estrogen-replacement therapy.[10,11] Because elevated estrogen increases the risk of breast and uterine cancer in women past menopause, this may be a matter of concern for those who wish to take supplemental boron. Further research is necessary to discover whether boron's apparent effects on estrogen is a real problem or not. At the present time, we would recommend getting your boron from fruits and vegetables: we know that they do not increase cancer risk (they reduce it).

⚠ Interactions You Should Know About

If you are receiving **hormone-replacement therapy**, use of boron may not be advisable due to the risk of elevating estrogen levels excessively.

CALCIUM

Supplement Forms/Alternate Names
Bonemeal, Calcium Aspartate, Calcium Carbonate, Calcium Chelate, Calcium Citrate, Calcium Citrate Malate, Calcium Gluconate, Calcium Lactate, Calcium Orotate, Dolomite, Oyster Shell Calcium, Tricalcium Phosphate

Principal Proposed Uses
Osteoporosis, PMS (Premenstrual Syndrome)

Other Proposed Uses
Colon Polyps and Cancer Prevention, Hypertension (High Blood Pressure), High Cholesterol, Attention Deficit Disorder, Migraine Headaches, Periodontal Disease, Preeclampsia

---

Calcium is the most abundant mineral in the body, making up nearly 2% of total body weight. More than 99% of the calcium in your body is found in your bones, but the other 1% is perhaps just as important for good health. Many enzymes depend on calcium in order to work properly, as do your nerves, heart, and blood-clotting mechanisms.

To build bone, you need to have enough calcium in your diet. But in spite of calcium-fortified orange juice and the best efforts of the dairy industry, most Americans are calcium deficient.[1] Calcium supplements are a simple way to make sure you're getting enough of this important mineral.

One of the most important uses of calcium is to prevent and treat osteoporosis, the progressive loss of bone mass to which postmenopausal women are especially vulnerable. Calcium works best when combined with vitamin D.

Recent evidence suggests that calcium may have another important use: dramatically reducing PMS symptoms.

Requirements/Sources

Although there are some variations between recommendations issued by different groups, the Adequate Intake for calcium is as follows

- Infants 0–6 months, 210 mg
  7–12 months, 270 mg
- Children 1–3 years, 500 mg
  4–8 years, 800 mg
- Males and females 9–18 years, 1,300 mg
  19–50 years, 1,000 mg
  51 years and older, 1,200 mg
- Pregnant women 1,000 mg (1,300 mg for females under 19 years old)
- Nursing women 1,000 mg (1,300 mg for females under 19 years old)

To absorb calcium, your body also needs an adequate level of vitamin D (for more information, see the chapter on vitamin D).

Milk, cheese, and other dairy products are excellent sources of calcium. Other good sources include orange juice or soy milk fortified with calcium, fish canned with its bones (e.g., sardines), dark green vegetables, nuts and seeds, and calcium-processed tofu.

If you wish to use calcium supplements, there are many forms available, each with its pros and cons. The most important ones include naturally derived forms of calcium, refined calcium carbonate, and chelated calcium.

Naturally Derived Forms of Calcium

These forms of calcium come from bone, shells, or the earth: bonemeal, oyster shell, and dolomite. Animals concentrate calcium in their shells, and calcium is found in minerals in the earth. These forms of calcium are economical, and you can get as much as 500 to 600 mg in one tablet. However, there are concerns that the natural forms of calcium supplements may contain significant amounts of lead.[2] Calcium supplements rarely list the lead content of their source, although they should. The lead concentration should always be less than 2 parts per million.

Refined Calcium Carbonate

This is the most common commercial calcium supplement, and it is also used as a common antacid. Calcium carbonate is one of the least expensive forms of calcium, but it can cause constipation and bloating, and it may not be well absorbed by people with reduced levels of stomach acid. Taking it with meals improves absorption, because stomach acid is released to digest the food.

Chelated Calcium

Chelated calcium is calcium bound to an organic acid (citrate, citrate malate, lactate, gluconate, aspartate, or orotate). The chelated forms of calcium offer some significant advantages and disadvantages compared with calcium carbonate.

On the plus side, certain forms of chelated calcium (calcium citrate and calcium citrate malate) appear to be better absorbed and more effective for osteoporosis treatment than calcium carbonate, although not all studies agree.[3-6] On the negative side, chelated calcium is much more expensive and bulkier than calcium carbonate. In other words, you have to take more and larger pills to get enough calcium. It is not at all uncommon to need to take five or six large capsules daily to supply the necessary amount, a quantity some people may find troublesome.

The form of calcium found in beverages is usually the chelated form, calcium citrate malate, or a slightly less well absorbed form, tricalcium phosphate.

Therapeutic Dosages

Unlike some supplements, calcium is not taken at extra high doses for special therapeutic benefit. Rather, for all its uses it should be taken in the amounts listed under Requirements/

Sources, along with the recommended level of vitamin D (see the chapter on vitamin D for proper dosage amounts).

Calcium absorption studies have found that your body can't absorb more than 500 mg of calcium at one time.[7] Therefore, it is most efficient to take your total daily calcium in two or more doses.

It isn't possible to put all the calcium you need in a single multivitamin/mineral tablet, so this is one supplement that should be taken on its own.

Furthermore, calcium may interfere with the absorption of chromium and manganese.[8,9,10] While it is sometimes stated that calcium can impair magnesium absorption, this does not appear to be the case.[11,12] Also, if you take any of these supplements, it is best to do so at a different time from when you take calcium. This means that it is best to take your multivitamin and mineral pill at a separate time from your calcium supplement.

Calcium may also interfere with iron absorption.[13–18] However, you shouldn't take extra iron unless you know you are deficient. (For more information, see the chapter on iron.)

While there is some evidence that calcium might decrease zinc absorption when the two are taken together, other studies disagree.[19–22] On balance, if there is any such effect at all, it must be slight.

Therapeutic Uses

There is little doubt that calcium supplementation is useful in helping prevent and slow down osteoporosis.[23–28]

If you are a woman past menopause, this is true whether or not you are taking estrogen. Calcium supplements work best when combined with vitamin D.

A new and rather surprising use of calcium came to light recently when a large, well-designed study found that calcium is an effective treatment for PMS (premenstrual syndrome).[29] Calcium supplementation reduced all major symptoms, including headache, food cravings, moodiness, and fluid retention. The benefits were so impressive that calcium should probably be considered the foremost treatment for PMS.

There may actually be a connection between these two uses of calcium: PMS may be an early sign of future osteoporosis.[30,31]

Recent evidence suggests that getting enough calcium may reduce the risk of developing colon cancer and colon polyps, a precancerous condition.[32]

Calcium deficiency appears to mildly increase blood pressure levels,[33,34] so if you have hypertension (high blood pressure), you should definitely make sure you get enough calcium.

Supplemental calcium appears to reduce total and LDL cholesterol by about 4% and raise HDL cholesterol by a similar amount.[35]

Calcium is also sometimes recommended for attention deficit disorder, migraine headaches, and periodontal disease, but there is as yet little to no evidence that it is effective.

Finally, calcium has been proposed as a treatment to prevent preeclampsia (a dangerous condition that can develop during pregnancy). However, a recent, very large, and well-designed study found it to be ineffective.[36]

What Is the Scientific Evidence for Calcium?

Osteoporosis

Numerous studies indicate that calcium supplements are useful in preventing and slowing osteoporosis, the progressive loss of bone mass as we age. Calcium supplementation at the recommended dosages appears to reduce bone loss in postmenopausal women in every part of the body except the spine.[37,38] When vitamin D is taken along with calcium, it may be possible not only to slow down but actually reverse osteoporosis, in the spine as well as in other bones.[39]

If you are taking estrogen to keep your bones strong, additional calcium may provide even more benefit.[40] Calcium supplementation is also useful for adolescent girls as a way to "put calcium in the bank"—building up a supply for the future.[41]

There is some good evidence that the use of calcium combined with vitamin D can help protect against the bone loss caused by corticosteroid drugs such as prednisone. In a 2-year, double-blind placebo-controlled study of 130 individuals, daily supplementation with 1,000 mg of calcium and 500 IU of vitamin D actually reversed steroid-induced bone loss, causing a net bone gain.[42]

Premenstrual Syndrome (PMS)

According to a large and well-designed study published in a 1998 issue of *American Journal of Obstetrics and Gynecology*, calcium supplements are a simple and effective treatment for a wide variety of PMS symptoms.[43] In a double-blind placebo-controlled study of 497 women, 1,200 mg daily of calcium as calcium carbonate reduced PMS symptoms by half over a period of three menstrual cycles. These symptoms included mood swings, headaches, food cravings, and bloating. These results corroborate earlier, smaller studies.[44,45]

Colon Cancer

Recent evidence suggests that the use of calcium carbonate can inhibit the development of precancerous polyps in the colon and rectum. A double-blind placebo-controlled study followed 832 individuals with a history of polyps for 4 years.[46] Participants received either 3 g daily of calcium carbonate or placebo. The calcium group experienced 24% fewer polyps overall than the placebo group.

There is also evidence from observational studies that a high calcium intake is associated with a reduced incidence of colon cancer,[47] but not all studies have found this association.[48]

Safety Issues

In general, it's safe to take up to 2,000 mg of calcium daily, although this is more than you need.[49] Greatly excessive intake of calcium can cause numerous side effects, including dangerous or painful deposits of calcium within the body.

If you have cancer, hyperparathyroidism, or sarcoidosis, you should take calcium only under a physician's supervision.

People with kidney stones or a history of kidney stones are also often warned not to take supplemental calcium. The reason for this caution is that kidney stones are commonly made of calcium oxalate crystals. However, studies have found that increased intake of calcium from food actually reduces the risk of kidney stones.[50,51] Calcium supplements, on the other hand, might increase kidney stone risk, especially if they are not taken with meals.[52] The bottom line? If you have a history of kidney stones, consult your physician before taking calcium supplements.

Large observational studies have found that higher intakes of calcium are associated with a greatly increased risk of prostate cancer.[53,54,55] This seems to be the case whether the calcium comes from milk or from calcium supplements. However, without further research it is difficult to tell whether this is a cause-and-effect relationship or simply an accidental correlation.

⚠ Interactions You Should Know About

If you are taking

- **Corticosteroids, heparin,** or **digoxin:** You may need more calcium.
- **Dilantin (phenytoin)** or **phenobarbital:** You may need more calcium; however, it may be advisable to take your dose of medication and your calcium supplement at least 2 hours apart because each interferes with the other's absorption.
- Antibiotics in the **tetracycline** or **fluoroquinolone** (Cipro, Floxin, Noroxin) families, or thyroid hormone: You should take your calcium supplement at least 2 hours before or after your dose of medication, because calcium interferes with the medications' absorption (and vice versa).
- **Thiazide diuretics** or **calcium channel-blockers:** Do not take extra calcium except on the advice of a physician.

- **Beta-blockers:** You should take calcium at least 2 hours before or after your medication.
- **Calcium:** You may need extra **iron, manganese, zinc,** and **chromium**. Ideally, you should take calcium at a different time of day from these other minerals, because it may interfere with their absorption.
- **Soy:** A constituent of soy called phytic acid can interfere with the absorption of calcium, so it may be advisable to wait 2 hours after taking calcium supplements to eat soy (or vice versa).

CARNITINE

Supplement Forms/Alternate Names
Acetyl-L-Carnitine (ALC), L-Acetyl-Carnitine (LAC), L-Carnitine,
L-Propionyl-Carnitine

Principal Proposed Uses
Angina and Other Heart Conditions, Intermittent Claudication,
Alzheimer's Disease, Depression in the Elderly

Other Proposed Uses
High Cholesterol, Performance Enhancement, Irregular Heartbeat,
Down's Syndrome, Muscular Dystrophy, Impaired Sperm Motility, Alcoholic Fatty Liver Disease, Toxicity Due to AZT (a Drug Used to Treat AIDS)
Chronic Obstructive Pulmonary Disease: Emphysema, Chronic Bronchitis

Carnitine is an amino acid the body uses to turn fat into energy. It is not normally considered an essential nutrient, because the body can manufacture all it needs. However, supplemental carnitine may improve the ability of certain tissues to produce energy. This effect has led to the use of carnitine in various muscle diseases as well as heart conditions.

Sources

There is no dietary requirement for carnitine. However, a few individuals have a genetic defect that hinders the body's ability to make carnitine. In addition, diseases of the liver, kidneys, or brain may inhibit carnitine production. Certain medications, especially the antiseizure drugs Depakene (valproic acid) and Dilantin (phenytoin), may reduce carnitine levels; however, whether taking extra carnitine would be helpful has not been determined.[1,2,3] Heart muscle tissue, because of its high energy requirements, is particularly vulnerable to carnitine deficiency.

The principal dietary sources of carnitine are meat and dairy products, but to obtain therapeutic dosages a supplement is necessary.

Therapeutic Dosages

Typical dosages for the diseases described here range from 500 to 1,000 mg 3 times daily. Carnitine is taken in three forms: L-carnitine (for heart and other conditions), L-propionyl-carnitine (for heart conditions), and acetyl-L-carnitine (for Alzheimer's disease). The dosage is the same for all three forms.

Therapeutic Uses

Carnitine is primarily used for heart-related conditions. Fairly good evidence suggests that it can be used along with conventional treatment for angina, or chest pain, to improve symptoms and reduce medication needs.[4-9] When combined with conventional therapy, it may also reduce mortality after a heart attack.[10,11]

Lesser evidence suggests that it may be helpful for a condition called intermittent claudication (pain in the legs after walking due to narrowing of the arteries),[12-20] as well as congestive heart failure.[21-24] Also a few studies suggest that carnitine may be useful for cardiomyopathy.[25,26]

Warning: You should not attempt to self-treat any of these serious medical conditions, nor should you use carnitine as a substitute for standard heart drugs.

Evidence also suggests that one particular form of carnitine, acetyl-L-carnitine, may be helpful in Alzheimer's disease,[27-33] although a recent large study found no benefit.[34] This form of carnitine may also be helpful for depression in the elderly.[35,36] Additionally, a preliminary study suggests that carnitine may be useful for individuals with type 2 (adult onset) diabetes.[37] Weak evidence suggests that carnitine may be able to improve cholesterol and triglyceride levels.[38]

Carnitine is widely touted as a physical performance enhancer, but there is no real evidence that it is effective and some research indicates that it does not work.[39] Little to no evidence supports other claimed benefits such as treating irregular heartbeat, Down's syndrome, muscular dystrophy, impaired sperm motility, chronic obstructive pulmonary disease (emphysema or chronic bronchitis), alcoholic fatty liver disease, and the toxicity of AZT (a drug used to treat AIDS).

What Is the Scientific Evidence for Carnitine?

Angina (Chest Pain)

Carnitine might be a good addition to standard therapy for angina. In one double-blind study, 200 individuals with angina (the exercise-induced variety) took either 2 g daily of L-carnitine or placebo. All the study participants continued to take their usual medication for angina. Those taking carnitine showed improvement in several measures of heart function, including a significantly greater ability to exercise without chest pain.[40] They were also able to reduce the dosage of some of their heart medications (under medical supervision) as their symptoms decreased. Similarly positive results were seen in another double-blind trial.[41]

Other studies using L-propionyl-carnitine have shown similar benefits.[42-45]

Intermittent Claudication

People with advanced hardening of the arteries, or atherosclerosis, often have difficulty walking due to lack of blood flow to the legs. Pain may develop after walking less than half a block. Although carnitine does not increase blood flow, it appears to improve the muscle's ability to function under difficult circumstances.[46] In a double-blind study of 245 individuals with intermittent claudication, those treated with 2 g daily of L-propionyl-carnitine showed a 73% improvement in walking distance.[47] This result is not quite as good as it sounds, because there was a 46% improvement with placebo (the power of suggestion is always amazing!), but it was nonetheless significant.

Similar results have been seen in most but not all other studies.[48–55] Interestingly, nearly all the studies on carnitine for this condition have been performed by one investigator. L-propionyl-carnitine seems to be more effective for intermittent claudication than plain carnitine.

For another approach, see the discussion of inositol hexaniacinate in the chapter on vitamin B_3.

Congestive Heart Failure

Several small studies have found that carnitine, often in the form of L-propionyl-carnitine, can improve symptoms of congestive heart failure.[56–59] However, there is better evidence for coenzyme Q_{10} for treating this condition.

After a Heart Attack

Carnitine may help reduce death rate after a heart attack. In a 12-month, placebo-controlled study, 160 individuals who had experienced a heart attack received 4 g of L-carnitine daily or placebo, in addition to other conventional medication. The mortality rate in the treated group was significantly lower than in the placebo group, 1.2% versus 12.5%, respectively. There were also improvements in heart rate, blood pressure, angina (chest pain), and blood lipids.[60] A larger double-blind study of 472 people found that carnitine may improve the chances of survival if given within 24 hours after a heart attack.[61]

Note: Carnitine is used along with conventional treatment, not as a substitute for it.

Alzheimer's Disease

Numerous double-blind or single-blind clinical studies involving a total of more than 1,400 people have evaluated the potential benefits of acetyl-L-carnitine in the treatment of Alzheimer's disease and other forms of dementia.[62–72] Most have found at least mildly positive results. However, the benefits are slight at most, and one of the best-designed studies found no benefit.

For example, one double-blind trial followed 130 individuals with mild to moderate Alzheimer's disease for 1 full year.[73] All participants worsened over that time, but according to 14 different measurements of mental function and behavior, the treated group deteriorated more slowly. However, the difference was not very large, and it was only statistically significant for a few of the rating scales used.

Some studies, however, have not found any benefit. In particular, a recent double-blind placebo-controlled trial that enrolled 431 participants for 1 year found no significant improvement at all in the group treated with acetyl-L-carnitine.[74]

The most likely explanation for the negative outcome in this well-designed study is that acetyl-L-carnitine produces only a small benefit at most.

Mild Depression

A double-blind study of 60 seniors with mild depression found that treatment with 3 g of carnitine daily over a 2-month period significantly improved symptoms as compared to placebo.[75] Positive results were seen in another study as well.[76]

Performance Enhancement

A 1996 review of clinical studies concluded that no scientific basis exists for the belief that carnitine supplements enhance athletic performance.[77] A few studies have found some benefit, but most have not.

Safety Issues

L-carnitine in its three forms appears to be safe, even when taken with medications. Individuals should take care, however, not to use forms of the supplement known as "D-carnitine" or

"DL-carnitine," as these can cause angina, muscle pain, and loss of muscle function (probably by interfering with L-carnitine).

The maximum safe dosages for young children, pregnant or nursing women, or those with severe liver or kidney disease have not been established.

⚠ Interactions You Should Know About

If you are taking antiseizure medications, particularly **valproic acid (Depakote, Depakene)** but also **phenytoin** (Dilantin), you may need extra carnitine.

CARTILAGE

Supplement Forms/Alternate Names
Bovine Cartilage, Shark Cartilage

Principal Proposed Uses
There are no well-documented uses for cartilage.

Other Proposed Uses
Cancer Treatment, Osteoarthritis, Psoriasis, Rheumatoid Arthritis

Cartilage is a tough connective tissue found in many parts of the body. Your ears and nose are made from cartilage, and so is the gliding surface in your joints.

One constituent of cartilage, chondroitin, is widely used in Europe to treat arthritis (for more information, see the chapter on chondroitin). Cartilage itself has also been proposed as a treatment for arthritis.

The most commonly used forms of cartilage come from cows (bovine cartilage) and sharks.

Shark cartilage contains chemical compounds that prevent new blood vessel growth in test-tube experiments. Because cancers must create new blood vessels to feed them, shark cartilage has been touted as a cure for cancer. However, there is no direct evidence that it works.

Sources

Unless your uncle works at a slaughterhouse or you're brave enough to prepare your own cartilage from whole sharks, the preferred source of cartilage is your health food store or pharmacy, where you can purchase this supplement in pill or powdered form.

Therapeutic Dosages

Various doses of cartilage have been used in different studies, ranging from 2.5 mg to 60 g daily.

Therapeutic Uses

Cartilage in general has been proposed as a treatment for the common "wear and tear" type of arthritis known as osteoarthritis. The idea behind this is straightforward: Because osteoarthritis is a disease of the joints, and because cartilage is one of the elements that make up your joints, adding cartilage to the diet might help. This idea sounds a bit too simplistic to be real, but it is the same principle behind the use of glucosamine and chondroitin for osteoarthritis, specific substances found in the joints. Since double-blind studies have found those treatments effective, perhaps cartilage itself will ultimately be proven to work. However, studies of cartilage have not yet been performed.

Cartilage has also been proposed for rheumatoid arthritis, again without any particular evidence that it works.

Shark cartilage in particular has been widely hyped as a cure for cancer. However, the evidence that it might work is so preliminary that drawing conclusions from the research available is like calling the results of an election 4 years before it happens based on one small public opinion poll. The science simply hasn't been done yet.

Based on very weak evidence, shark cartilage has also been suggested as a treatment for psoriasis.[1]

What Is the Scientific Evidence for Cartilage?

There is no good clinical evidence yet that cartilage can cure or relieve symptoms of any disease.

A number of test-tube experiments have found that shark cartilage extracts prevent new blood vessels from forming in chick embryos and other test systems.[2,3,4] Developing drugs to prevent blood vessels from forming in tumors is an exciting new approach to treating cancer. Unfortunately, we don't have any research data on human subjects, so we can't say whether shark cartilage really has any effect on tumors in human beings. More study is needed.

Safety Issues

Because cartilage is just common, ordinary gristle, it is presumably safe to consume.

CHONDROITIN

Supplement Forms/Alternate Names
Chondroitin Sulfate
Principal Proposed Uses
Osteoarthritis
Other Proposed Uses
Atherosclerosis, High Cholesterol

Chondroitin sulfate is a naturally occurring substance in the body. It is a major constituent of cartilage—the tough, elastic connective tissue found in the joints.

Based on the evidence of preliminary double-blind studies, chondroitin is widely used in Europe as a treatment for osteoarthritis, the "wear and tear" arthritis that many people suffer as they get older.

Furthermore, chondroitin may go beyond treating symptoms and actually protect joints from damage. Current medical treatments for osteoarthritis, such as NSAIDs (nonsteroidal anti-inflammatory drugs), treat the symptoms but don't actually slow the disease's progression, and they may actually make it worse faster.[1-5] Chondroitin (along with glucosamine and SAMe) may take the treatment of osteoarthritis to a new level. However, more research needs to be performed to prove definitively that this exciting possibility is real.

Sources

Chondroitin is not an essential nutrient. Animal cartilage is the only dietary source of chondroitin. (When it's on your plate, animal cartilage is called gristle.) Unless you enjoy chewing gristle, you'd do best to obtain chondroitin in pill form from a health food store or pharmacy.

Therapeutic Dosages

The usual dosage of chondroitin is 400 mg taken 3 times daily. Be patient! The results take weeks to develop. In commercial products it is often combined with glucosamine. Preliminary information from one animal study suggests that this combination may be superior to either treatment alone.[6]

Therapeutic Uses

Initially, chondroitin was primarily used in an injectable form. But in recent years, double-blind studies using the oral form of chondroitin for osteoarthritis have been reported.[7,8,9] The best evidence is for a pain-relieving effect, but some studies have found that it can also slow the progression of the disease.[10–13]

Chondroitin has also been proposed as a treatment for other conditions such as atherosclerosis and high cholesterol, but as yet the evidence that it might help is quite preliminary.[14,15]

What Is the Scientific Evidence for Chondroitin?

For years, experts stated that oral chondroitin couldn't possibly work, because its molecules are so big that it seemed doubtful that they could be absorbed through the digestive tract. However, in 1995 researchers laid this objection to rest when they found evidence that up to 15% of chondroitin is absorbed intact.[16]

Reducing Symptoms of Osteoarthritis

Three recently published double-blind placebo-controlled studies involving a total of about 250 participants suggest that chondroitin can relieve symptoms of osteoarthritis. One enrolled 85 people with osteoarthritis of the knee and followed them for 6 months.[17] Participants received either 400 mg of chondroitin sulfate twice daily or placebo. At the end of the trial, doctors rated the improvement as good or very good in 69% of those taking chondroitin sulfate but in only 32% of those taking placebo.

Another way of comparing the results is to look at maximum walking speed among participants. Whereas individuals in the chondroitin group were able to improve their walking speed gradually over the course of the trial, walking speed did not improve at all in the placebo group. Additionally, there were improvements in other measures of osteoarthritis, such as pain level, with benefits seen as early as 1 month. This suggests that chondroitin was able to stop the arthritis from gradually getting worse (see also Slowing the Progression of Osteoarthritis).

Similar results were found in another study that was shorter (3 months) but followed more individuals (127 people).[18]

A third double-blind study involved only 42 participants; however, it followed them for a full year.[19] Chondroitin took months to reach its full effect but eventually relieved symptoms considerably better than placebo.

Positive results were also seen in earlier studies, including one that found chondroitin about as effective as the anti-inflammatory drug dicloflenac.[20-23]

Slowing the Progression of Osteoarthritis

An interesting feature of the full-year study mentioned previously was that, whereas the placebo group showed progressive joint damage over the year, no worsening of the joints was seen in the group taking chondroitin. In other words, chondroitin seemed to protect the joints from damage, thus slowing or perhaps even halting the progression of the disease. Osteoarthritis tends to get worse with time.

As mentioned earlier, no conventional treatment for osteoarthritis protects joints from progressive damage, and some may actually accelerate the process. If further studies confirm that chondroitin prevents progressive damage to the joints, it would make chondroitin distinctly better than any conventional option. Unfortunately, this study was too small to prove anything on its own.

Another, larger study examined the progression of osteoarthritis in 119 people for 3 full years.[24] In this double-blind placebo-controlled trial, those who took 1,200 mg of chondroitin daily showed lower rates of severe joint damage. Only 8.8% of the chondroitin group developed severely damaged joints during the 3 years of the study, compared with almost 30% of the placebo group. This suggests that chondroitin was slowing the progression of osteoarthritis. Unfortunately, the researchers did not report whether this difference was statistically significant.

Additional evidence comes from animal studies. The effect of both oral and injected chondroitin was assessed in rabbits with damaged cartilage in the knee.[25] After 84 days of treatment, the rabbits that were given chondroitin had significantly more healthy cartilage remaining in the damaged knee than the untreated animals. Receiving chondroitin by mouth was as effective as taking it through an injection.

Putting all this information together, it appears quite likely that chondroitin can slow the progression of osteoarthritis. However, more studies are needed to confirm this very exciting possibility. It would also be wonderful if chondroitin could repair damaged cartilage and thus reverse arthritis, but none of the research so far shows such an effect. Chondroitin may simply stop further destruction from occurring.

How Does Chondroitin Work for Osteoarthritis?

Scientists are unsure how chondroitin sulfate works, but one of several theories (or all of them) might explain its mode of action.

At its most basic level, chondroitin may help cartilage by providing it with the building blocks it needs to repair itself. It is also believed to block enzymes that break down cartilage in the joints.[26,27] Another theory holds that chondroitin increases the amount of hyaluronic acid in the joints.[28] Hyaluronic acid is a protective fluid that keeps the joints lubricated. Finally, chondroitin may have a mild anti-inflammatory effect.[29]

Safety Issues

Chondroitin sulfate has not been associated with any serious side effects, which is not surprising when you consider that taking it by mouth is essentially the same as eating gristle. Subjects in clinical trials have found mild digestive distress to be the only real complaint.

CHROMIUM

Supplement Forms/Alternate Names
Chromium Chloride, Chromium Picolinate, Chromium Polynicotinate, High-Chromium Brewer's Yeast
Principal Proposed Uses
Diabetes, Weight Loss
Other Proposed Uses
High Cholesterol and Triglycerides, Syndrome X, Functional Hypo-glycemia, Acne, Migraine Headaches, Psoriasis

Chromium is a mineral the body needs in very small amounts, but it plays an important role in human nutrition. Most of us are more familiar with chromium's industrial uses—for example, to make chrome-plated steel. Chromium's role in maintaining good health was discovered in 1957, when scientists extracted a substance known as glucose tolerance factor (GTF) from pork kidney. GTF, which helps the body maintain normal blood sugar levels, contains chromium.

Chromium's most important function is to help regulate the amount of glucose (sugar) in the blood. Insulin plays a starring role in this fundamental biological process, by regulating the movement of glucose out of the blood and into cells. Scientists believe that insulin uses chromium as an assistant (technically, a cofactor) to "unlock the door" to the cell membrane, thus allowing glucose to enter the cell.

Based on chromium's close relationship with insulin, this trace mineral has been studied as a treatment for diabetes. The results have been positive: chromium supplements appear to improve blood sugar control in people with diabetes.

Recent evidence also suggests that chromium supplements might help dieters lose fat and gain lean muscle tissue.

Requirements/Sources

No Recommended Dietary Allowance has been established for chromium, but the Estimated Safe and Adequate Daily Dietary Intake is as follows

- Infants under 6 months, 10 to 40 mcg
  6 months to 1 year, 20 to 60 mcg
- Children 1 to 3 years, 20 to 80 mcg
  4 to 6 years, 30 to 120 mcg
- Adults (and children 7 years and older), 50 to 200 mcg

Many Americans may be chromium-deficient.[1] Preliminary research done by the U.S. Department of Agriculture (USDA) in 1985 found low chromium intakes in a small group of people studied. Although large-scale studies are needed to show whether Americans as a whole are chromium deficient, we do know that many traditional sources of chromium, such as wheat, are depleted of this important mineral during processing.

Some researchers believe that inadequate intake of chromium may be one of the causes of the rising rates of adult-onset diabetes. However, the matter is greatly complicated by the fact that we lack a good test to determine chromium deficiency.[2]

Severe chromium deficiency has only been seen in hospitalized individuals receiving nutrition intravenously. Symptoms include problems with blood sugar control that cannot be corrected by insulin alone.

Chromium is found in drinking water, especially hard water, but concentrations vary so widely throughout the world that drinking water is not a reliable source. The most concentrated sources of chromium are brewer's yeast (not nutritional or torula yeast) and calf liver. Two ounces of brewer's yeast or 4 ounces of calf liver supply between 50 and 60 mcg of chromium. Other good sources of chromium are whole-wheat bread, wheat bran, and rye bread. Potatoes, wheat germ, green pepper, and apples offer modest amounts of chromium.

Calcium carbonate interferes with the absorption of chromium.[3]

Therapeutic Dosages

The dosage of chromium used in studies ranges from 200 to 1,000 mcg daily. However, there may be potential risks in the higher dosages of chromium (see Safety Issues).

Therapeutic Uses

Chromium has principally been studied for its possible benefits in improving blood sugar control in people with diabetes. Reasonably good evidence suggests that people with adult-onset (type 2) diabetes may show some improvement when given appropriate dosages of chromium.[4] One study suggests that chromium may be useful for diabetes that occurs during pregnancy.[5] Chromium also appears to help treat subtle problems with blood sugar control that are too mild to deserve the name "diabetes" but may cause an increased risk of heart disease.[6,7]

Recent evidence suggests that chromium supplements may also help reduce fat in the body, probably through its effects on insulin,[8] although not all studies have found positive results.[9]

Weak and contradictory evidence suggests that chromium may lower cholesterol and triglyceride levels.[10,11] In individuals taking beta-blockers, chromium may raise levels of HDL ("good") cholesterol.[12]

According to some authorities, impaired blood sugar control, high cholesterol, weight gain, and high blood pressure are all part of a bigger picture, given the mysterious-sounding name Syndrome X. Since chromium may be helpful for the first three of these conditions, chromium deficiency has been proposed as the cause of Syndrome X. However, the entire concept of Syndrome X is controversial, and many experts don't believe that it even exists.

Chromium is often suggested as a treatment for the opposite of diabetes, hypoglycemia (low blood sugar). In reality, this condition may not involve lower-than-normal levels of blood sugar at all but rather an abnormal response to normal changes in blood sugar levels. Possible symptoms include anxiety, sweating, and shakiness, which may develop between meals and are relieved by eating. However, there is no direct evidence that chromium is effective for this condition.

Chromium has also been proposed as a treatment for acne, migraine headaches, and psoriasis, but there is as yet no real evidence that it works.

What Is the Scientific Evidence for Chromium?

Diabetes

Moderately strong evidence supports the use of chromium for diabetes. In a recent, double-blind placebo-controlled study, 180 people with type 2 diabetes were given either placebo, 200 mcg of chromium picolinate daily, or a higher dosage of chromium picolinate—1,000 mcg daily. Individuals taking 1,000 mcg showed marked improvements in blood sugar levels. Lesser but still significant benefits were also seen in the 200-mcg group but not in the placebo group.[13]

Similarly positive results were seen in other small studies.[14,15] However, there have also been negative results.[16]

One double-blind study of 30 women with pregnancy-related diabetes found that supplementation with chromium (at a dosage of 4 or 8 mcg chromium picolinate for each kilogram of body weight) significantly improved blood sugar control.[17]

Improved Blood Sugar Control in People Without Diabetes

Numerous small studies have found that chromium supplementation can improve mild abnormalities in blood sugar control,[18,19,20] although one study found no benefit.[21] There is growing evidence that mildly impaired blood sugar control increases the risk of heart disease. Chromium supplementation may be appropriate.

Weight Loss

Recent evidence suggests that chromium may be an effective aid in weight loss.

A 3-month double-blind study of 122 moderately overweight individuals attempting to lose weight found that 400 mcg of chromium daily resulted in an average loss of 6.2 pounds of body fat, as opposed to 3.4 pounds in the placebo group. There was no loss of lean body mass.[22] These results suggest that chromium can help you lose body fat without losing muscle. It may work by helping the body process its insulin more effectively.

However, in one small double-blind placebo-controlled study, chromium picolinate at a dose of 400 mcg actually led to weight gain in young obese women.[23] When combined with exercise training, chromium picolinate produced no net effect. Interestingly, 400 mcg of chromium nicotinate combined with exercise did induce weight loss.

Safety Issues

Chromium appears to be safe when taken at a dosage of 50 to 200 mcg daily.[24] Side effects appear to be rare.

However, chromium is a heavy metal and might conceivably build up and cause problems if taken to excess. There is one report of kidney damage in a person who took 1,200 to 2,400 mcg of chromium for several months; in another report, as little as 600 mcg for 6 weeks was enough to cause damage.[25,26]

For this reason, the dosage found most effective for individuals with type 2 diabetes—1,000 mcg daily—might present some health risks. It would be advisable to seek medical supervision if you want to take more than 200 mcg daily.

Also, keep in mind that if you have diabetes and chromium is effective, you may need to cut down your dosage of any medication you take for diabetes. Medical supervision is advised.

There has been one report of a severe skin reaction caused by chromium picolinate.[27]

Concerns have also been raised over the use of the picolinate form of chromium in individuals suffering from affective or psychotic disorders, because picolinic acids can change the levels of neurotransmitters.[28] There are also concerns, still fairly theoretical, that chromium picolinate could cause adverse effects on DNA.[29]

The maximum safe dosages of chromium for young children, women who are pregnant or nursing, or those with severe liver or kidney disease have not been established.

⚠ Interactions You Should Know About

If you are taking

- **Calcium carbonate supplements** or **antacids:** You may need extra chromium. You should also separate your chromium supplement and your doses of these substances by at least 2 hours, because they may interfere with chromium's absorption.
- **Oral diabetes medications** or **insulin:** Seek medical supervision before taking chromium because you may need to reduce your dose of these medications.
- **Beta-blockers:** Chromium supplementation may improve levels of HDL ("good") cholesterol.

COENZYME Q$_{10}$ (CoQ$_{10}$)

Supplement Forms/Alternate Names
Ubiquinone
Principal Proposed Uses
Congestive Heart Failure, Cardiomyopathy, Other Forms of Heart Disease, Hypertension, Nutrient Depletion Caused by Various Medications
Other Proposed Uses
Periodontal Disease, Male Infertility, AIDS, Cancer, Obesity, Muscular Dystrophy, Enhanced Performance for Athletes

Coenzyme Q10 (CoQ$_{10}$), also known as ubiquinone, is a powerful antioxidant discovered by researchers at the University of Wisconsin in 1957. The name of this supplement comes from the word *ubiquitous*, which means "found everywhere." Indeed, CoQ$_{10}$ is found in every cell in the body. It plays a fundamental role in the mitochondria, the parts of the cell that produce energy from food.

Japanese scientists first discovered the therapeutic properties of CoQ$_{10}$ in the 1960s. Today, it is widely prescribed for heart conditions in Europe and Israel, as well as in Japan. CoQ$_{10}$ appears to assist the heart during times of stress on the heart muscle, perhaps by helping it use energy more efficiently. While CoQ$_{10}$'s best-established use is for congestive heart failure, ongoing research suggests that it may also be useful for other types of heart problems and for a wide variety of additional illnesses.

Sources

Every cell in your body needs CoQ$_{10}$, but no U.S. Recommended Dietary Allowance has been established for this important substance because the body can manufacture CoQ$_{10}$ from scratch.

Because CoQ$_{10}$ is found in all animal and plant cells, we obtain small amounts of this nutrient from our diet. However, it would be hard to get a therapeutic dosage from food.

Therapeutic Dosages

The typical recommended dosage of CoQ_{10} is 30 to 300 mg daily, often divided into 2 or 3 doses. CoQ_{10} is fat soluble and is better absorbed when taken in an oil-based soft gel form rather than in a dry form such as tablets and capsules.[1]

Therapeutic Uses

The best-documented use of CoQ_{10} is for treating congestive heart failure.[2–5] Keep in mind that it is taken along with conventional medications, not instead of them.

Weaker evidence suggests that it may be useful for cardiomyopathy and other forms of heart disease.[6,7,8] CoQ_{10} has been suggested as a treatment for hypertension[9–12] and to prevent the heart damage caused by certain types of cancer chemotherapy. Keep in mind that CoQ_{10} might conceivably interfere with the action of other chemotherapy drugs (although there is no good evidence that it does so). Therefore, if you are a cancer patient, check with your oncologist before using CoQ_{10}.

CoQ_{10} is sometimes claimed to be an effective treatment for periodontal disease. However, the studies on which this idea is based are too flawed to be taken as meaningful.[13] CoQ_{10} has additionally been proposed as a treatment for a wide variety of other conditions, including angina, male infertility, AIDS, cancer, obesity, and muscular dystrophy. It has also been used as a performance enhancer for athletes. However, as yet the evidence to support these uses remains weak.

CoQ_{10} has become popular as a treatment for possible nutritional depletion caused by various medications. It has been suggested (but not proven) that CoQ_{10} deficiency may play a role in the known side effects of these treatments, and that taking CoQ_{10} supplements might be a good idea.

The best evidence is for the cholesterol-lowering drugs in the statin family, such as lovastatin (Mevacor), simvastatin (Zocor), and pravastatin (Pravachol).[14,15,16]

For several other categories of drugs, the evidence that they cause depletion of CoQ$_{10}$ is fairly indirect. These include oral diabetes drugs (especially glyburide, phenformin, and tolazamide), beta-blockers (specifically propranolol, metoprolol, and alprenolol), antipsychotic drugs in the phenothiazine family, tricyclic antidepressants, methyldopa, hydrochlorothiazide, clonidine, and hydralazine.[17–21]

What Is the Scientific Evidence for Coenzyme Q$_{10}$ (CoQ$_{10}$)?

Congestive Heart Failure

Very good evidence tells us that CoQ$_{10}$ can be helpful for people with congestive heart failure (CHF). In this serious condition, the heart muscles become weakened, resulting in poor circulation and shortness of breath.

People with CHF have significantly lower levels of CoQ$_{10}$ in heart muscle cells than healthy people.[22] This fact alone does not prove that CoQ$_{10}$ supplements will help CHF; however, it prompted medical researchers to try using CoQ$_{10}$ as a treatment for heart failure.

The results have been positive. At least nine double-blind studies have found that CoQ$_{10}$ supplements can markedly improve symptoms and objective measurements of heart function when they are taken along with conventional medication.

In the largest of these studies, 641 individuals with moderate to severe congestive heart failure were monitored for 1 year.[23] Half were given 2 mg per kilogram body weight of CoQ$_{10}$ daily; the rest were given placebo. Standard therapy was continued in both groups. The participants treated with CoQ$_{10}$ experienced a significant reduction in the severity of their symptoms. No such improvement was seen in the placebo group. The people who took CoQ$_{10}$ also had significantly fewer hospitalizations for heart failure.

Similarly positive results were also seen in smaller studies involving a total of over 300 participants.[24,25,26]

Cardiomyopathy

Cardiomyopathy is the general name given to conditions in which the heart muscle gradually becomes diseased. Several small studies suggest that CoQ_{10} supplements are helpful for some forms of cardiomyopathy.[27,28,29]

Hypertension

An 8-week, double-blind placebo-controlled study of 59 men already taking medications for high blood pressure found that 120 mg daily of CoQ_{10} could reduce blood pressure by about 9% as compared to placebo.[30]

Similar results were seen in other trials, most of which were not double-blind.[31,32,33]

An interesting feature of the 8-week study described previously is that use of CoQ_{10} led to improvements in insulin and blood sugar levels, suggesting additional benefits in the treatment of diabetes.

Safety Issues

CoQ_{10} appears to be extremely safe. No significant side effects have been found, even in studies that lasted a year.[34] However, individuals with severe heart disease should not take CoQ_{10} (or any other supplement) except under a doctor's supervision.

The maximum safe dosages of CoQ_{10} for young children, pregnant or nursing women, or those with severe liver or kidney disease have not been determined.

⚠ Interactions You Should Know About

If you are taking

- **Cholesterol-lowering drugs** in the statin family, **beta-blockers** (specifically **propranolol**, **metoprolol**, and **alprenolol**), antipsychotic drugs in the **phenothiazine** family, **tricyclic antidepressants**, **methyldopa**, **hydrochlorothiazide**, **clonidine**, or **hydralazine:** You may need more coenzyme Q_{10}.

- **Oral diabetes drugs** (especially **glyburide**, **phenformin**, and **tolazamide**): You may need more coenzyme Q_{10}. However, it's possible that coenzyme Q_{10} could reduce your blood sugar levels, requiring a decrease in medication.

COLOSTRUM

Principal Proposed Uses
Prevention of Infections
Other Proposed Uses
Ulcer Prevention

Colostrum is the fluid that new mothers' breasts produce during the first day or two after birth. It gives newborn infants a rich mixture of antibodies and growth factors that help them get a good start.

Although colostrum has been available since the first mammals walked the earth, it is relatively new as a nutritional supplement. The resurgence of breastfeeding in the 1970s sparked a revival of interest in colostrum for both infants and adults. However, most commercial colostrum preparations come from cows, not humans. Whether cow antibodies are good for humans is unclear. Colostrum primarily fights gastrointestinal infections, but a cow's digestive tract is so different from yours and mine that benefits may not cross over.

Requirements/Sources

Breastfeeding is the healthiest way to nourish a newborn, and a mother's colostrum is undoubtedly good for a baby. But don't believe claims (by at least one manufacturer) that most babies would die without colostrum. Colostrum is good for health, but it's not essential for life.

Colostrum has just become available in capsules that contain its immune proteins in dry form.

Therapeutic Dosages

The usual recommended dosage of colostrum is 10 g daily.

Therapeutic Uses

Colostrum is often sold as an "immune stimulant." However, if it works at all, it should function by directly fighting microorganisms. There is no particular reason to believe it would strengthen your immune system. In any case, while some studies have found it effective against viruses or parasites, about as many have found it ineffective.[1–6]

For years, people with ulcers were advised to drink a bland diet with lots of milk. Although this treatment was eventually found to be ineffective, it does seem that colostrum (although not milk) might help protect the stomach from damage caused by anti-inflammatory drugs, at least according to one study in rats.[7]

What Is the Scientific Evidence for Colostrum?

Preventing Infections

There is some evidence that colostrum can help in certain infectious diseases, but other studies have found it ineffective. Several highly preliminary studies indicate that colostrum may relieve diarrhea and other symptoms associated with Cryptosporidium in people with AIDS.[8,9] However, in another study, colostrum failed to produce a significant effect on Cryptosporidium infection.[10]

Another study suggests that colostrum might help prevent infections with the Shigella parasite.[11] However, a different study looking at Bangladeshi children infected with *Helicobacter pylori* (the organism that causes digestive ulcers) found no benefits.[12] Also, no benefit was seen in a study on rotavirus (another parasite that causes diarrhea in children).[13]

Safety Issues

Colostrum does not seem to cause any significant side effects. However, comprehensive safety studies have not been performed. Safety in young children or women who are pregnant or nursing has not been established.

CONJUGATED LINOLEIC ACID

Supplement Forms/Alternate Names
CLA

Principal Proposed Uses
There are no well-documented uses for conjugated linoleic acid.

Other Proposed Uses
Reducing Body Fat

Conjugated linoleic acid (CLA) is a mixture of different isomers, or chemical forms, of linoleic acid. This is an essential fatty acid—a type of fat that your body needs as much as it needs vitamins. Although it has become popular as a "fat-burning" supplement, we don't really know how or even whether CLA really works.

Requirements/Sources

Although linoleic acid itself is an important nutritional source of essential fatty acids, there is no evidence that you need to get *conjugated* linoleic acid in your diet. CLA does occur in food, but it would be very difficult to get the recommended dose that way. Supplements are the only practical source.

Therapeutic Dosages

The typical dosage of CLA ranges from 3 to 5 g daily. As with all supplements taken at this high a dosage, it is important to purchase a reputable brand, as even very small amounts of a toxic contaminant could quickly mount up.

Therapeutic Uses

There is some evidence that CLA might help you lose fat while retaining muscle. However, what we know is based primarily on some interesting animal studies and very small human clinical trials.[1,2] Better studies in humans are currently under way, but results are not currently available. At present, there is more evidence that chromium can provide this benefit (for more information, see the chapter on chromium).

Safety Issues

CLA appears to be a safe nutritional substance. However, maximum safe dosages for young children, pregnant or nursing women, or those with severe liver or kidney disease have not been determined.

COPPER

Supplement Forms/Alternate Names
Copper Complexes of Various Amino Acids, Copper Gluconate, Copper Picolinate, Copper Sulfate

Principal Proposed Uses
There are no well-documented uses for copper.

Other Proposed Uses
Osteoporosis, High Cholesterol, Heart Disease, Osteoarthritis, Rheumatoid Arthritis

The human body contains only 70 to 80 mg of copper, but it's an essential part of many important enzymes. Copper's possible role in treating disease is based on the fact that these enzymes can't do their jobs without it. However, there is little direct evidence that taking extra copper can treat any disease.

Requirements/Sources

Although a precise dietary requirement for copper has not been determined, the Estimated Safe and Adequate Daily Dietary Intake is as follows

- Infants under 6 months, 0.4 to 0.6 mg
    6 months to 1 year, 0.6 to 0.7 mg
- Children 1 to 3 years, 0.7 to 1.0 mg
    4 to 6 years, 1.0 to 1.5 mg
    7 to 10 years, 1.0 to 2.0 mg
    11 to 18 years, 1.5 to 2.5 mg
- Adults 19 years and older, 1.5 to 3.0 mg

Marginal copper deficiency appears to be common in Western diets.[1] Excessive zinc intake reduces copper stores in the body.[2]

Oysters, nuts, legumes, whole grains, sweet potatoes, and dark greens are good sources of copper. Drinking water that passes through copper plumbing is a good source of this mineral, and sometimes it may even provide too much.

Therapeutic Dosages

The typical adult supplemental dosage of copper is 1 to 3 mg daily.

Therapeutic Uses

Copper has been proposed as a treatment for osteoporosis, based primarily on studies that found benefit using mixtures of various trace minerals.[3,4]

One researcher, L. M. Klevay, has claimed in more than a dozen papers that copper deficiencies increase the risk of high cholesterol and heart disease, but he has failed to supply any real evidence that this idea is true. A double-blind clinical trial of copper supplements for reducing heart disease risk found no benefit.[5]

Similarly, copper has long been mentioned as a possible treatment for osteoarthritis and rheumatoid arthritis, but there is as yet no real evidence that it works.

Safety Issues

Copper is safe when taken at nutritional dosages, but these should not be exceeded. As little as 10 mg of copper daily produces nausea, and 60 mg may cause vomiting. Maximum

safe dosages of copper for young children, pregnant or nursing women, or those with severe liver or kidney disease have
not been determined.

⚠ Interactions You Should Know About

If you are taking

- **Zinc:** You need to make sure to get enough copper.
- **Iron** supplements, **manganese**, or high doses of **vitamin C:** You may need extra copper. If you do take a
  copper supplement, it might be ideal to take it either 2
  hours before or after these other substances.[6]
- **Oral contraceptives:** It might not be advisable to
  take extra copper.
- **Copper:** You may need extra manganese.

CREATINE

Supplement Forms/Alternate Names
Creatine Monohydrate

Principal Proposed Uses
Exercise Performance Involving High-Intensity, Short-Term Bursts
of Activity

Other Proposed Uses
Weight Loss, Improved Ratio of Body Fat to Muscle, High Triglycerides,
Amyotrophic Lateral Sclerosis (ALS, Lou Gehrig's Disease), Huntington's
Disease, Congestive Heart Failure, Mitochondrial Illnesses

Creatine is a naturally occurring substance that plays an important role in the production of energy in the body. The
body converts it to phosphocreatine, a form of stored energy
used by muscles.

In recent years, many athletes have tried supplemental
creatine as a performance enhancer. If you're a U.S. baseball
fan, you probably know that Mark McGwire, the all-time single-season home run champ, takes creatine (along with many
other supplements).

Although the evidence for creatine is not definitive, of all sports supplements, it has the most evidence behind it. Numerous small double-blind studies suggest that it can increase athletic performance in sports that involve intense but short bursts of activity.

The theory behind its use is that supplemental creatine can build up a reserve of phosphocreatine in the muscles, to help them perform on demand. Supplemental creatine may also help the body make new phosphocreatine faster when it has been used up by intense activity.

Sources

Although some creatine exists in the daily diet, it is not an essential nutrient because your body can make it from the amino acids L-arginine, glycine, and L-methionine. Provided you eat enough protein (the source of these amino acids), your body will make all the creatine you need for good health.

Meat (including chicken and fish) is the most important dietary source of creatine and its amino acid building blocks. For this reason, vegetarian athletes may potentially benefit most from creatine supplementation.

Therapeutic Dosages

For bodybuilding and exercise enhancement, a typical dosage schedule starts with a "loading dose" of 15 to 30 g daily (divided into 2 or 3 separate doses) for 3 to 4 days, followed by 2 to 5 g daily. Some authorities recommend skipping the loading dose. (By comparison, we typically get only about 1 g of creatine in the daily diet.)

Creatine's ability to enter muscle cells can be increased by combining it with glucose, fructose, or other simple carbohydrates. Caffeine appears to block the effects of creatine.[1]

Therapeutic Uses

Creatine is one of the bestselling and best-documented supplements for enhancing athletic performance, but the scientific evidence that it works is far from complete. The best evidence we have points to benefits in forms of exercise that require repeated short-term bursts of high-intensity exercise, such as soccer and basketball.[2,3,4]

Creatine has also been proposed as an aid to promote weight loss and to reduce the proportion of fat to muscle in the body, but there is little evidence that it is effective for this purpose.[5] Better evidence exists for chromium in this regard.

Preliminary evidence suggests that creatine supplements may be able to reduce levels of triglycerides in the blood.[6] (Triglycerides are fats related to cholesterol that also increase risk of heart disease when elevated in the body.)

Preliminary studies, including small double-blind trials, suggest that creatine may be helpful for various muscle illnesses, including amyotrophic lateral sclerosis (Lou Gehrig's disease), congestive heart failure, Huntington's disease, and mitochondrial illnesses.[7–15] Although the evidence is still not strong, creatine seems to be able to reduce fatigue and increase strength in these conditions.

What Is the Scientific Evidence for Creatine?

Exercise Performance

Several small double-blind studies suggest that creatine can improve performance in exercises that involve repeated short bursts of high-intensity activity.[16]

For example, in one double-blind study, 16 physical education students exercised 10 times for 6 seconds on a stationary cycle, alternating with a 30-second rest period.[17] The results showed that individuals who took 20 g of creatine for 6 days were better able to maintain cycle speed. Similar results were seen in many other studies.[18,19,20]

Isometric exercise capacity (pushing against a fixed resistance) also seems to improve with creatine.[21]

However, studies of endurance or nonrepeated exercise have *not* shown benefits.[22,23,24] Therefore, creatine probably won't help you for marathon running or single sprints.

High Triglycerides

A 56-day, double-blind placebo-controlled study of 34 men and women found that creatine supplementation can reduce levels of triglycerides in the blood by about 25%.[25] Effects on other blood lipids such as total cholesterol were insignificant.

Safety Issues

Creatine appears to be safe, at least in healthy athletes. No significant side effects have been found with the regimen of several days of a high dosage (15 to 30 g daily) followed by 6 weeks of a lower dosage (2 to 3 g daily). We do not know whether it is safe to use creatine for longer periods.

Two deaths have been reported in individuals taking creatine, but other causes were most likely responsible.[26] Although fears have been expressed about creatine causing kidney injury, evidence suggests that creatine is safe for people whose kidneys are healthy to begin with, and who don't take excessive doses.[27] However, individuals with kidney disease, especially those on dialysis, should probably avoid creatine.

As with all supplements taken in very high doses, it is important to purchase a high-quality form of creatine, as contaminants present even in very low concentrations could conceivably build up and cause problems.

DHEA (DEHYDROEPIANDROSTERONE)

Supplement Forms/Alternate Names
DHEA Sulfate

Principal Proposed Uses
Lupus, Adrenal Failure

Other Proposed Uses
Osteoporosis, Slowing Aging, Improving General Well-Being, Depression, Impotence, Alzheimer's Disease, Chronic Fatigue Syndrome, Sports Performance

Dehydroepiandrosterone (DHEA), a hormone produced by the adrenal glands, is the most abundant hormone in the steroid family found in the bloodstream. Your body uses DHEA as the starting material for making the sex hormones testosterone and estrogen.

Numerous popular books have made extravagant claims about DHEA, but in reality we know very little about the effects of DHEA supplements. A growing number of physicians have begun to report that DHEA is helpful for the autoimmune disease lupus, but the evidence is as yet preliminary. DHEA does appear to be helpful when taken along with standard treatment for adrenal failure. Keep in mind that DHEA is not a natural supplement. The DHEA you can buy at the store is made by a synthetic chemical process, and it is a hormone, not a nutrient. Although DHEA appears to be safe to use in the short term, its safety when taken for prolonged periods is unknown.

Sources

The body makes its own DHEA; we get very little in our diets. DHEA production peaks early in life and begins to decline as we reach adulthood. By age 60, our bodies produce just 5 to 15% as much as when we were 20. It's not clear whether this decline in DHEA is a bad thing, but some believe that it may contribute to the aging process.

For use as a dietary supplement, DHEA is manufactured synthetically from substances found in soybeans. Contrary to popular belief, there is no DHEA in wild yam.

Therapeutic Dosages

A typical therapeutic dosage of DHEA is 50 to 200 mg daily, although some studies used dosages above and below this range. A cream containing 10% DHEA may also be used; it is typically applied to the skin at a dosage of 3 to 5 g daily.

Physicians sometimes check DHEA levels and adjust the daily dose to achieve blood levels of 20 to 30 nmol/L.

Therapeutic Uses

Preliminary evidence suggests that DHEA might help reduce symptoms of lupus.[1,2] This is an area of active study at present, and may result in a new approach to treating this chronic autoimmune disease.

A very small study (14 participants) suggests that DHEA cream (10%, 3 to 5 g daily) can help fight osteoporosis.[3] Anti-osteoporosis benefits were also seen in a study of individuals with severe lupus.[4]

Primarily because DHEA decreases with age, this hormone has been widely hyped as a kind of fountain of youth. However, there is no real evidence that taking DHEA will slow down any of the effects of aging. In fact, it is perfectly possible that DHEA levels decrease for some health-promoting reason. In addition, one study found that DHEA supplementation does not increase general well-being in healthy people.[5]

In some individuals, the adrenal glands fail to work, typically due to illness (or surgical removal of the adrenal glands). Traditionally, such people are given a variety of hormonal medications to make up for what their own adrenal glands are not producing. These hormones preserve the lives of individuals with adrenal failure, but they don't completely restore health. This may be due to the fact that the normal adrenal gland makes DHEA, a hormone not usually supplied in standard treatment. One double-blind study of women with adrenal failure found that adding DHEA supplements to the usual treatment improved feelings of well-being, sexual function, and even cholesterol levels.[6] Although this study was small, it was published in a major journal and will likely influence medical practice.

However, keep in mind that the vague concept of "adrenal weakness," widely discussed in natural medicine circles, is not the same as adrenal failure, and there is no reason to believe that DHEA would make a difference in those circumstances.

DHEA is also sometimes suggested for depression on the basis of one small double-blind study and one observational study.[7,8]

A small double-blind study suggests that DHEA might be helpful for men who find it difficult to achieve an erection, when blood tests show they are low in this hormone.[9]

Highly preliminary evidence suggests that DHEA might be helpful for chronic fatigue syndrome.[10]

There are good theoretical reasons (but little direct evidence) to believe that individuals taking corticosteroids (such as prednisone) might be protected from some of the side effects by taking DHEA at the same time.[11,12]

Although DHEA is sometimes recommended as a sports supplement, what evidence there is suggests that it does not work.[13,14]

DHEA has also been proposed for Alzheimer's disease, although as yet there is little evidence to support this use.

What Is the Scientific Evidence for DHEA?

Lupus

A preliminary double-blind placebo-controlled study suggests that DHEA may be helpful for treating symptoms of the serious autoimmune disease lupus.[15] However, this study was too small (only 28 participants) to mean a great deal on its own. Possible benefits were seen in another small study as well.[16] Larger studies are presently under way.

Adrenal Insufficiency

A study published in the *New England Journal of Medicine* supports adding DHEA to the usual hormone regimen for adrenal failure.[17] This double-blind placebo-controlled trial evaluated the effects of DHEA in 24 women with adrenal insufficiency. The results showed that DHEA improved sexual function, feelings of overall well-being, and cholesterol levels.

Impotence

A double-blind placebo-controlled study enrolled 40 men with difficulty achieving or maintaining an erection, who also had low measured levels of DHEA.[18] The results showed that DHEA at a dose of 50 mg daily significantly improved sexual performance.

Sports Performance

A small double-blind study found no benefit with DHEA at a dose of 150 mg per day for men undergoing weight training.[19] In addition, a 12-week, double-blind study of 40 trained male athletes given either DHEA or androstenedione at 100 mg daily found no improvement in lean body mass or strength, or change in testosterone levels.[20]

Safety Issues

DHEA appears to be safe when taken in therapeutic doses, at least in the short term. One study found no significant side effects in 50 women who took up to 200 mg daily for up to 1 year.[21] However, other studies suggest that DHEA may cause acne, male pattern hair growth, and decreased levels of HDL cholesterol.[22]

Concerns have been raised by one study in rats and another in trout that linked DHEA to liver cancer.[23,24] However, at least four other animal studies suggest that DHEA may have some anticancer effects.[25,26]

The long-term safety of DHEA is entirely unknown. This is the case with many supplements, but because there are animal studies suggesting that DHEA might increase the risk of liver cancer, caution is warranted. Estrogen is one example of a hormone that increases the risk for certain forms of cancer, and it took years for researchers to discover that risk. Keep in mind also that the body converts DHEA into other hormones, including estrogen. This effect could be dangerous for women with hormone-influenced diseases such as breast cancer.

The safety of DHEA in young children, pregnant or nursing women, and individuals with severe liver or kidney disease has not been established. We also don't know whether DHEA interacts with other hormone treatments, such as estrogen, although it certainly stands to reason that it might.

⚠ Interactions You Should Know About

If you are taking **corticosteroids** (such as prednisone), you might be protected from some side effects by taking DHEA at the same time.

FISH OIL

Supplement Forms/Alternate Names
Docosahexaenoic Acid (DHA), Eicosapentaenoic Acid (EPA), Omega-3 Fatty Acids, Omega-3 Oil(s)

Principal Proposed Uses
Heart Disease Prevention, Rheumatoid Arthritis

Other Proposed Uses
Dysmenorrhea (Menstrual Pain), Bipolar Disease (Manic-Depressive Illness), Raynaud's Phenomenon, Psoriasis, Osteoporosis, Lupus, Crohn's Disease, Depression, Prevention of Premature Birth, Vision Improvement in Premature Babies, Diabetic Neuropathy, Allergies, Gout, Hypertension, Migraine Headaches, Ulcerative Colitis, Asthma

---

If you're old enough, you may remember your mother giving you cod liver oil. This practice actually began when the smoke-filled skies of nineteenth-century England deprived youngsters of exposure to the sun. Without sun, their bodies couldn't make vitamin D, and they developed rickets. Because cod liver oil contains large amounts of vitamin D, it cured rickets and made a great contribution to public health. Today, however, other constituents of cod liver and other fish oils have become of interest: the omega-3 fatty acids.

Omega-3 fatty acids are one type of *essential fatty acids*, special fats that the body needs as much as it needs vitamins. (The other type is the omega-6 fatty acids. For more information, see the chapter on GLA.) Much of the research into the potential therapeutic benefits of omega-3 fatty acids began when studies of the Inuit (Eskimo) people found that although their diets contain an enormous amount of fat from fish, seals, and whales, they seldom suffer heart attacks or develop rheumatoid arthritis. This is presumably because those sources of fat are very high in omega-3 fatty acids.

Subsequent investigation found that the omega-3 fatty acids found in fish oil can lower blood triglyceride levels, "thin" the blood, and also decrease inflammation in various parts of the body. These effects, as well as others, may explain many of fish oil's apparent benefits.

Requirements/Sources

There is no daily requirement for fish oil. However, a healthy diet should provide at least 5 g of essential fatty acids daily.

Many grains, fruits, vegetables, and vegetable oils contain significant amounts of essential omega-6 and/or omega-3 fatty acids. Some authorities believe that it is important to consume several times more omega-3 fatty acids than omega-6 fatty acids. If this theory is true, taking fish oil supplements might help ensure the proper balance.

Cod liver oil is the most common form of fish oil, but it may not be the best for reasons of safety (see Safety Issues). Salmon oil, mackerel oil, halibut oil, and the oils from other coldwater fish might be better choices.

Therapeutic Dosages

Typical dosages of fish oil are 3 to 9 g daily, but this is not the upper limit. In one study, participants ingested 60 g daily.

The most important omega-3 fatty acids found in fish oil are called EPA (eicosapentaenoic acid) and DHA (docosahexacnoic acid). In order to match the dosage used in several major studies, you should probably take enough fish oil to supply about 1.8 g of EPA (1,800 mg) and 0.9 g of DHA daily (900 mg).

Some manufacturers add vitamin E to fish oil capsules to keep the oil from becoming rancid. Another method is to remove all the oxygen from the capsule.

Flaxseed oil also contains omega-3 fatty acids, although of a different kind. It has been suggested as a less smelly substitute for fish oil. However, there is no evidence that it is effective when used for the same therapeutic purposes as fish oil.[1]

Therapeutic Uses

There has been a great deal of excitement about the possibility of using fish oil to help prevent heart disease. Fish or fish oil appears to lower triglyceride levels, raise HDL ("good") cholesterol, "thin" the blood, reduce levels of homocysteine, slow down atherosclerosis, and perhaps also treat hypertension.[2–13]

Fish oil has also become recognized as an effective treatment for early stages of rheumatoid arthritis. It appears to significantly reduce symptoms without side effects and may magnify the benefits of standard arthritis drugs.[14] However, we have no evidence that fish oil slows the progress of the disease. Consult your rheumatologist to determine what treatment is best for you.

Various essential fatty acids, including fish oil, flaxseed oil, and GLA (gamma-linolenic acid), are widely recommended for dysmenorrhea (menstrual pain), and a study of adolescent women suggests that fish oil may indeed be effective.[15]

A study suggests that fish oil can be very helpful for bipolar disease, more commonly known as manic-depressive disorder.[16] More research is needed, but this appears to be a potential breakthrough for this devastating illness, whose conventional treatment causes a great many side effects.

Small studies also suggest that fish oil may be helpful in Raynaud's phenomenon (a condition in which a person's hands and feet show abnormal sensitivity to cold temperatures),[17,18] psoriasis,[19] osteoporosis,[20,21] the autoimmune disease lupus,[22] and Crohn's disease.[23]

Interesting, but highly preliminary, evidence suggests that fish oil, or its constituents, might be helpful for treating depression, preventing premature birth, and improving vision in premature babies.[24,25,26]

Fish oil has also been proposed as a treatment for many other conditions, including diabetic neuropathy,[27] allergies, gout, migraine headaches, and ulcerative colitis, but there has been little real scientific investigation of these uses. Fish oil does not appear to be helpful for asthma, and one study found that it can actually worsen aspirin-related asthma.[28,29,30]

What Is the Scientific Evidence for Fish Oil?

Heart Disease Prevention

There is some evidence that fish oil can help prevent heart disease, but it is not definitive.

An open trial of 11,324 individuals followed for 3 to 5 years did find that fish oil could significantly reduce the risk of death from heart attack, and that it was more effective for this purpose than vitamin E.[31] However, because this was not a double-blind study, the results can't be taken as fully reliable.

We do know that fish oil can lower serum triglycerides.[32] Like cholesterol, triglycerides are a type of fat in the blood that tends to damage the arteries, leading to heart disease. Reducing triglyceride levels should help prevent heart disease to some extent.

Fish oil also appears to modestly raise the levels of HDL ("good") cholesterol.[33,34] Additionally, it may help the heart by "thinning" the blood and by reducing blood levels of homocysteine.[35] Blood clots play a major role in heart attacks, and homocysteine is an amino acid that appears to raise the risk of heart disease.

Studies contradict one another on whether fish oil can lower blood pressure.[36–41] A 6-week, double-blind placebo-controlled study of 59 overweight men suggests that the DHA in fish oil, but not the EPA, can reduce blood pressure.[42]

Rheumatoid Arthritis

The omega-3 fatty acids in fish oil can help reduce the symptoms of rheumatoid arthritis, according to 12 double-blind placebo-controlled studies involving a total of over 500 people.[43] This evidence is so strong that it has impressed many conventional physicians. However, unlike some conventional treatments, fish oil probably does not slow the progression of rheumatoid arthritis.

Menstrual Pain

Regular use of fish oil may reduce the pain of menstrual cramps. In a 4-month study of 42 young women aged 15 to

18, half the participants received a daily dose of 6 g of fish oil, providing 1,080 mg of EPA and 720 mg of DHA daily.[44] After 2 months, they were switched to placebo for another 2 months. The other group received the same treatments in reverse order.

The results showed that these young women experienced significantly less menstrual pain while they were taking fish oil.

Bipolar Disease

A 4-month, double-blind placebo-controlled study of 30 individuals suggests that fish oil can produce striking benefits in bipolar disease, preventing relapse and improving emotional state.[45] Eleven of the 14 individuals who took fish oil improved or remained well during the course of the study, while only 6 out of the 16 given placebo responded similarly.

The study will now be repeated by Baylor University and Harvard Medical School/McLean Hospital, enrolling 120 people for a period of 3 years.

Raynaud's Phenomenon

In small double-blind studies, high dosages of fish oil have been found to reduce the severe finger and toe responses to cold temperatures that occur in Raynaud's phenomenon.[46,47] However, these studies suggest that a very high dosage must be used to get results, perhaps 12 g daily. Gamma-linolenic acid (GLA), an omega-6 fatty acid, may work as well.

Psoriasis

There is some evidence that eicosapentaenoic acid (EPA) from fish oil may be helpful in psoriasis. One double-blind study followed 28 people with chronic psoriasis for 8 weeks.[48] Half received 1.8 g of EPA daily (supplied by 10 capsules of fish oil), and the other half received placebo. By the end of the study, researchers saw significant improvement in itching, redness, and scaling, but not in the size of the psoriasis patches. However, another double-blind study followed 145 people with moderate to severe psoriasis for 4 months and found no benefit as compared to placebo.[49]

Osteoporosis

Essential fatty acids may also help prevent osteoporosis when taken along with calcium. In one study, 65 postmenopausal women were given calcium along with either placebo or a combination of omega-6 fatty acids (GLA) and omega-3 fatty acids (from fish oil) for a period of 18 months. At the end of the study, the treated groups had denser bones and fewer fractures than the placebo group.[50] Similar results were seen in another study of 40 women.[51]

Lupus

Lupus is a serious autoimmune disease that can cause numerous problems, including fatigue, joint pain, and kidney disease. One small, 34-week, double-blind placebo-controlled crossover study compared placebo against daily doses of EPA (20 g) from fish oil.[52] A total of 17 individuals completed the trial. Of these, 14 showed improvement when taking EPA, while only 4 did so when treated with placebo.

Safety Issues

Fish oil appears to be safe. The most common problem is fishy burps.

Because fish oil has a mild "blood-thinning" effect, it should not be combined with powerful blood-thinning medications, such as Coumadin (warfarin) or heparin, except on a physician's advice. However, contrary to some reports, fish oil does not seem to cause bleeding problems when it is taken by itself.[53]

Also, fish oil does not appear to raise blood sugar levels in people with diabetes.[54] Nonetheless, if you have diabetes, you should not take any supplement except on the advice of a physician.

Fish oil may temporarily raise the level of LDL ("bad") cholesterol, but this effect seems to be short-lived, and levels return to normal with continued use.[55,56]

If you decide to use cod liver oil as your fish oil supplement, make sure you do not exceed the safe maximum intake of vitamin A and vitamin D. These vitamins are fat soluble, which means that excess amounts tend to build up in your body, possibly reaching toxic levels. Pregnant women should not take more than 2,667 IU of vitamin A daily because of the risk of birth defects; 5,000 IU per day is a reasonable upper limit for other individuals. Look at the bottle label to determine how much vitamin A you are receiving. (It is less likely that you will get enough vitamin D to produce toxic effects.)

⚠ Interactions You Should Know About

If you are taking **Coumadin (warfarin)** or **heparin**, do not take fish oil except on the advice of a physician.

FLAXSEED OIL

Supplement Forms/Alternate Names
Linseed Oil
Principal Proposed Uses
There are no well-documented uses for flaxseed oil.
Other Proposed Uses
Heart Disease Prevention, Rheumatoid Arthritis, Cancer Prevention
Note: Flaxseed oil contains alpha-linolenic acid.

Flaxseed oil is derived from the hard, tiny seeds of the flax plant. It has been proposed as a less smelly alternative to fish oil. Like fish oil, flaxseed oil contains omega-3 fatty acids, a type of fat your body needs as much as it needs vitamins.

However, it's important to realize that the omega-3 fatty acids in flaxseed oil aren't identical to what you get from fish oil. Flaxseed oil contains alpha-linolenic acid (ALA), while fish oil contains eicosapentaenoic acid (EPA) and docosahexaenoic acid (DHA). The effects and potential benefits may not be the same.

Flaxseeds contain another important group of chemicals known as *lignans*. Lignans are being studied for use in preventing cancer. However, contrary to some reports, flaxseed *oil* has no lignans.[1]

Requirements/Sources

Flaxseed oil contains both omega-3 and omega-6 fatty acids, which are essential to health. Although the exact daily requirement of these essential fatty acids is not known, deficiencies are believed to be fairly common.[2] Flaxseed oil may be an economical way to ensure that you get enough essential fatty acids in your diet.

The essential fatty acids in flax can be damaged by exposure to heat, light, and oxygen (essentially, they become rancid). For this reason, you shouldn't cook with flaxseed oil. A good product should be sold in an opaque container, and the manufacturing process should keep the temperature under 100 degrees Fahrenheit. Some manufacturers combine the product with vitamin E because it helps prevent rancidity.

Therapeutic Dosages

A typical dosage is 1 to 2 tablespoons of flaxseed oil daily. It can be taken in capsule form or made into salad dressing. Some people find the taste pleasant, although others would politely disagree.

For whole flaxseed, a typical dose is 1 tablespoon of the seed (not ground) with plenty of liquid 2 to 3 times daily.

Therapeutic Uses

The best use of flaxseed oil is as a general nutritional supplement to provide essential fatty acids. There is little evidence that it is effective for any specific therapeutic purpose.

Flaxseed oil has been proposed as a less smelly alternative to fish oil for the prevention of heart disease. Although fish oil is much better studied, there is some evidence that flaxseed oil or whole flaxseed may reduce LDL ("bad") cholesterol, perhaps slightly reduce hypertension, and, overall, slow down atherosclerosis.[3,4,5]

In addition, one study found that a diet high in ALA (from sources other than flaxseed oil) was associated with a reduced risk of heart disease.[6] However, there were so many other factors involved that it is hard to say what caused what.[7]

Although fish oil appears to be effective for reducing symptoms of rheumatoid arthritis, flaxseed oil does not seem to work.[8]

Finally, although flaxseed or flaxseed oil are sometimes recommended as prevention or treatment for cancer, the evidence is still extremely preliminary.[9–12]

Safety Issues

Flaxseed oil appears to be a safe nutritional supplement when used as recommended.

FOLATE

Supplement Forms/Alternate Names
Folacin, Folic Acid

Principal Proposed Uses
Prevention of Birth Defects of the Brain and Spinal Cord, Heart Disease Prevention, Cancer Prevention

Other Proposed Uses
Gout, Bipolar Disorder, Depression, Osteoarthritis, Osteoporosis, Restless Legs Syndrome, Rheumatoid Arthritis, Vitiligo, Migraine Headaches, Periodontal Disease

Folate, a B vitamin, plays a critical role in many biological processes. It participates in the crucial biological process known as methylation, and plays an important role in cell division: without sufficient amounts of folate, cells cannot divide properly. Adequate folate intake can reduce the risk of heart disease and prevent serious birth defects, and it may lessen the risk of developing certain forms of cancer.

Because the chances are good that you don't get enough folate in your diet, this is one vitamin really worth paying attention to.

Requirements/Sources

Folate requirements rise with age. The U.S. Recommended Dietary Allowance is as follows

- Infants under 6 months, 25 mcg
  6 to 12 months, 35 mcg
- Children 1 to 3 years, 150 mcg
  4 to 8 years, 200 mcg
- Males 9 to 13 years, 300 mcg
  14 years and older, 400 mcg
- Females 9 to 13 years, 300 mcg
  14 years and older, 400 mcg
- Pregnant women, 600 mcg
- Nursing women, 500 mcg

Folate deficiency is very common, and authorities have suggested adding folate to common foods, such as bread, at higher dosages than what is presently required.[1,2]

Various drugs may impair your body's ability to absorb or utilize folate, including antacids, bile acid sequestrants (such as cholestyramine and colestipol), estrogen, H_2 blockers, methotrexate, various antiseizure medications (carbamazepine, phenobarbital, phenytoin, primidone, or valproate), sulfasalazine and possibly other certain NSAID-type drugs, and the antibiotic trimethoprim-sulfamethoxazole.[3-10] Oral contraceptives may also affect folate, but the evidence is not consistent.[11-15]

Good sources of folate include dark green leafy vegetables, oranges, other fruits, rice, brewer's yeast, beef liver, beans, asparagus, soybeans, and soy flour.

Therapeutic Dosages

For most uses, folate should be taken at nutritional doses, about 400 mcg daily for adults. However, higher dosages— up to 10 mg daily—have been used to treat specific diseases. Before taking more than 400 mcg daily, it is important to make sure that you don't have a vitamin B_{12} deficiency (see Safety Issues).

A particular kind of digestive enzyme, pancreatin (see the chapter on proteolytic enzymes) may interfere with the absorption of folate.[16] You can get around this by taking the two supplements at different times of day.

Therapeutic Uses

The use of folate supplements by pregnant women dramatically decreases the risk that their children will be born with a serious birth defect called neural tube defect.[17,18] This congenital problem consists of problems with the brain or spinal cord.

Folate also lowers blood levels of homocysteine, a suspected risk factor in heart disease.[19–24] According to some experts, increased folate supplementation of foods could reduce heart disease deaths in the United States by as much as 50,000 people annually.[25]

Studies suggest that a deficiency in folate might predispose people to develop cancer of the cervix,[26] colon,[27] lung,[28] breast,[29] and mouth.[30] This is yet another reason to make sure you get enough folate daily. High-dose folate (10 mg daily) might be helpful for normalizing abnormalities in the appearance of the cervix (as seen under a microscope) in women taking oral contraceptives, but it does not appear to reverse actual cervical dysplasia.[31,32]

Very high dosages of folate may also be helpful for gout,[33] although some authorities suggest that it was actually a contaminant of folate that caused the benefit seen in some studies.[34] Furthermore, other studies have found no benefit at all.[35,36]

Based on intriguing but not yet definitive evidence, folate in various dosages has been suggested as a treatment for bipolar disorder, depression, osteoarthritis (in combination with vitamin B_{12}), osteoporosis, restless legs syndrome, rheumatoid arthritis, and vitiligo (splotchy loss of skin pigmentation).[37–47] Other conditions for which it has been suggested include migraine headaches and periodontal disease.

What Is the Scientific Evidence for Folate?

Neural Tube Defect

Very strong evidence tells us that regular use of folate by pregnant women can reduce the risk of neural tube defect by 50 to 80%.[48,49]

Heart Disease Prevention

According to a recent study that examined data on 80,000 women, a high intake of folate may cut the risk of heart disease in half.[50]

Folate is thought to work by reducing blood levels of a substance called homocysteine. Individuals with high homocysteine levels appear to have more than twice the risk of developing heart disease than those with low homocysteine levels,[51] and folate supplements, alone or in combination with vitamin B_6 and vitamin B_{12}, effectively reduce the level of homocysteine in the blood.[52–55]

Safety Issues

Folate at nutritional doses is extremely safe. The only serious potential problem is that folate supplementation can mask the early symptoms of vitamin B_{12} deficiency (a special type of anemia), potentially allowing more irreversible symptoms of nerve damage to develop. For this reason, when taking more than 400 mcg daily, it is important to get your B_{12} level checked. See the chapter on vitamin B_{12} for more information.

Very high dosages of folate, greater than 5 mg (5,000 mcg) daily, can cause digestive upset. According to a few reports, folate can occasionally cause an increase of seizures in those with epilepsy and may interfere with the antiseizure drug phenytoin.[56,57]

Maximum safe dosages have not been established for young children or pregnant or nursing women.

Contrary to some reports, individuals who are taking the drug methotrexate for rheumatoid arthritis, juvenile rheumatoid arthritis, or psoriasis can safely take folate supplements at the same time.[58,59,60] However, if you are taking methotrexate for any other purpose, do not take folate except on the advice of a physician.

⚠ Interactions You Should Know About

If you are taking

- Aspirin, other anti-inflammatory medications, drugs that reduce stomach acid (such as antacids and H_2 blockers), sulfa antibiotics, oral contraceptives, estrogen-replacement therapy, valproic acid, carbamazepine, phenobarbital, primidone, nitrous oxide, or **bile acid sequestrants (such as cholestyramine and colestipol):** You may need to take extra folate.
- **Phenytoin:** You may need more folate. However, too much folate can interfere with this medication and cause seizures! Physician supervision is essential.
- **Pancreatin** (a proteolytic enzyme): You should take folate at a different time of day to avoid absorption problems.
- **Methotrexate** for rheumatoid arthritis, juvenile rheumatoid arthritis, or psoriasis: You may do well to take a folate supplement. You can use folate without fear of decreasing the medication's effects. However, if you are taking methotrexate for other purposes, do not take folate except on the advice of a physician.

GAMMA ORYZANOL

Principal Proposed Uses
Menopausal Symptoms ("Hot Flashes"), High Cholesterol
Other Proposed Uses
Anxiety, Stomach Distress, Bodybuilding

Gamma oryzanol is a mixture of substances derived from rice bran oil, including sterols and ferulic acid. It has been approved in Japan for several conditions, including menopausal symptoms, mild anxiety, stomach upset, and high cholesterol. Each year Japan manufactures 7,500 tons of gamma oryzanol from 150,000 tons of rice bran. Not surprisingly, most of the research on oryzanol has been performed in Japan and few studies have been translated into English.

Scientists are not certain how gamma oryzanol works. For menopause, it may affect a key hormone, luteinizing hormone (LH). Gamma oryzanol may also interfere with the absorption of cholesterol into the body from food, thus reducing cholesterol levels in the blood.

Sources

There is no daily requirement for gamma oryzanol.

Rice bran oil is the principal source of gamma oryzanol, but it is also found in the bran of wheat and other grains, as well as various fruits, vegetables, and herbs. However, to get enough gamma oryzanol to reach recommended therapeutic dosages, you will need to take supplements.

Therapeutic Dosages

The typical dosage of gamma oryzanol is 300 mg daily.

Therapeutic Uses

Despite the widespread use of gamma oryzanol for menopausal symptoms, the studies available in English provide little evidence that it is effective. The most commonly cited Japanese study was very small and did not have a control group.[1]

Gamma oryzanol may be useful for elevated cholesterol, although the evidence is highly preliminary.[2,3] No serious evidence has been presented in English for using gamma oryzanol as a treatment for anxiety or stomach distress.

Very preliminary evidence suggests that gamma oryzanol may increase endorphin release and aid muscle development.[4,5] These findings have created an interest in using gamma oryzanol as a sports supplement. However, one double-blind study found it not effective.[6]

What Is the Scientific Evidence for Gamma Oryzanol?

Menopausal Symptoms

Gamma oryzanol may be effective in treating hot flashes associated with menopause. An early study examined 21 women, 8 who were experiencing menopause and 13 who had had their ovaries surgically removed. Each woman was given 300 mg daily of gamma oryzanol.[7] After 38 days, more than 67% of the women improved significantly. However, because this study had no control group, there's no way to know whether the benefit was caused by gamma oryzanol or merely the power of suggestion. Keep in mind that at least 50% of menopausal women given placebo experience significant relief from symptoms.[8]

High Cholesterol

The best evidence that gamma oryzanol can lower cholesterol levels comes from animal studies. In one such study, 32 hamsters with experimentally induced high cholesterol were given a high-saturated–fat diet containing 5% coconut oil and 0.1% cholesterol, with or without 1% oryzanol, for 7 weeks.[9] Despite the unhealthy diet, the hamsters that were given oryzanol absorbed 25% less cholesterol from their food than the control group, and experienced a significant (28%) drop in total cholesterol in the blood. A small, uncontrolled study in people found similar reductions in cholesterol.[10]

Bodybuilding

A 9-week, double-blind placebo-controlled trial of 22 weight-trained males found no difference between placebo or 500 mg daily of gamma oryzanol in terms of performance, body composition, or hormone levels.[11]

Safety Issues

No significant side effects have been reported with gamma oryzanol. However, the maximum safe dosages for young children, pregnant or nursing women, or those with severe liver or kidney disease have not been established.

GLA (GAMMA-LINOLENIC ACID)

Supplement Forms/Alternate Names
Omega-6 Fatty Acids, Omega-6 Oil(s), Sources of GLA include Black Currant Seed Oil, Borage Oil, Evening Primrose Oil
Principal Proposed Uses
Cyclic Mastalgia (Cyclic Mastitis, Fibrocystic Breast Disease, Mastodynia), General PMS Symptoms, Diabetic Neuropathy, Eczema
Other Proposed Uses
Rheumatoid Arthritis, Raynaud's Phenomenon, Osteoporosis, Asthma, and Many Others

GLA (gamma-linolenic acid) is one of the two main types of *essential fatty acids*. These are "good" fats that are as necessary for your health as vitamins. Specifically, GLA is an omega-6 fatty acid. (For more information on the other major category of essential fatty acids, omega-3, see the chapter on fish oil.)

The body uses essential fatty acids to make various prostaglandins and leukotrienes. These substances influence inflammation and pain; some of them increase symptoms, while others decrease them. Taking GLA may swing the balance over to the more favorable prostaglandins and leukotrienes, making it helpful for diseases that involve inflammation.

GLA is widely used in Europe to treat diabetic neuropathy and eczema. Both European and U.S. physicians use GLA to treat cyclic mastalgia, a condition marked by breast pain associated with the menstrual cycle. It may also be useful for other PMS symptoms.

GLA has also been proposed as a treatment for many other conditions.

Requirements/Sources

The body ordinarily makes all the GLA it needs from linoleic acid, an omega-6 essential fatty acid found in many foods. In certain circumstances, however, the body may not be able to convert linoleic acid to GLA efficiently. These include advanced age, diabetes, high alcohol intake, eczema, cyclic mastitis, viral infections, excessive saturated fat intake, elevated cholesterol levels, and deficiencies of vitamin B_6, zinc, magnesium, biotin, or calcium.[1–5] In such cases, taking GLA supplements may make up for a genuine deficiency.

Very little GLA is found in the diet. Borage oil is the richest supplemental source (17 to 25% GLA), followed by black currant oil (15 to 20%) and evening primrose oil (7 to 10%). Borage and evening primrose are the most common sources.

Therapeutic Dosages

The usual dosage of GLA used to treat cyclic mastalgia or eczema is about 200 to 400 mg daily (about 2 to 4 g of evening primrose oil or 1 to 2 g of borage oil). Diabetic neuropathy is typically treated with about 400 to 600 mg daily (about 4 to 6 g of evening primrose or 2 to 3 g of borage oil), and rheumatoid arthritis may require as much as 2,000 to 3,000 mg (best obtained from purified GLA).

GLA should be taken with food. Don't forget that full benefits may take over 6 months to develop, so be patient.

Therapeutic Uses

Most commonly in the form of evening primrose oil, GLA has become a standard treatment for cyclic mastalgia, breast pain that cycles with the menstrual period.[6–9] It is widely used for this purpose by conventional physicians in both Europe and North America, and as a mark of its acceptance it is even mentioned in the AMA's official *Drug Evaluations* textbook.[10]

Evening primrose oil is also said to be useful for other PMS symptoms, although the evidence is not strong.[11]

Evening primrose oil also appears to be effective for diabetic neuropathy,[12,13] a complication of diabetes. This condition, which develops in many people with diabetes, consists of pain and/or numbness due to progressive nerve damage.

Additionally, evening primrose oil is widely used in Europe as a treatment for eczema. Unfortunately, scientific evidence suggesting that it works is mixed at best, and the most recent studies have not found it to be effective.[14–18]

Very high doses of purified GLA may be of some benefit in treating rheumatoid arthritis, especially when combined with conventional treatments.[19–22] GLA may also help in Raynaud's phenomenon (a condition in which the fingers and toes react to cold in an exaggerated way)[23,24] as well as osteoporosis.[25,26]

Thus far, we've mentioned only a fraction of the conditions for which GLA has been proposed as a treatment. Others include asthma, allergies, bursitis, chronic fatigue syndrome, endometriosis, heart disease, irritable bowel syndrome, prostate cancer, prostate enlargement or benign prostatic hyperplasia (BPH), Sjogren's disease, and many more. However, none of these potential uses has as yet any strong evidence behind it.

One double-blind study found that evening primrose oil is not helpful for weight loss.[27]

What Is the Scientific Evidence for GLA (Gamma-Linolenic Acid)?

Cyclic Mastalgia

Cyclic mastalgia, also known as fibrocystic breast disease, cyclic mastitis, and mastodynia, is a condition in which a woman's breasts become painful during the week or two before her menstrual period. The discomfort is accompanied by swelling, inflammation, and sometimes actual cysts that form in the breasts. It is often associated with other symptoms of premenstrual syndrome (PMS).

We do not know the cause of cyclic mastalgia, but researchers have found that it seems to be associated with an imbalance of fatty acids in the body.[28]

Evidence suggests that GLA relieves cyclic mastalgia, perhaps by restoring the balance of essential fatty acids.[29] One report published in 1985 compares the effectiveness of four different therapies in women with severe, painful mastalgia: GLA from evening primrose oil and the pharmaceuticals danazol, bromocriptine, and progestins (often, but not quite accurately, called progesterone).[30]

The results suggest that evening primrose oil was effective in just under 50% of participants. However, this was not actually a study in the usual sense; it was more a collation of records from the Cardiff Clinic, a medical center that specializes in the treatment of breast pain. Contrary to how this study is sometimes reported, it did not have a placebo group.

To really know whether a treatment is effective, you need double-blind placebo-controlled studies to eliminate the power of suggestion. One such study was reported in 1981. This trial followed 73 women suffering from cyclic mastalgia.[31] The results were consistent with the Cardiff Clinic's results, finding that evening primrose oil reduced pain in almost 50% of the women taking it, while only 19% of the women improved in the placebo group.

However, this study was reported only in a very brief form, and many details are missing. We really need better designed and better reported studies to know for sure how effective evening primrose oil is for cyclic mastalgia.

If you have a severe form of cyclic mastalgia with actual breast cysts, there is some evidence that evening primrose oil will not be completely effective. In a double-blind study of 200 women treated for 1 year, evening primrose oil had no effect on recurrent breast cysts.[32,33] The conclusion appears to be that evening primrose oil relieves breast pain but cannot make breast cysts go away.

Other PMS Symptoms

Although several small studies suggest that GLA as evening primrose oil is helpful in reducing overall PMS symptoms, all of them suffer from serious flaws.[34]

Diabetic Neuropathy

Diabetic neuropathy is a gradual degeneration of nerves caused by diabetes. There is some evidence that GLA can be helpful, if you give it long enough to work. In one double-blind placebo-controlled study, 111 people with mild diabetic neuropathy received either 480 mg daily of GLA or placebo.[35] After 12 months, the group taking GLA was doing significantly better than the placebo group. Good results were seen in a smaller study as well.[36]

In addition, numerous studies in animals have found that evening primrose oil can protect nerves from diabetes-induced nerve injury.[37,38]

GLA may work especially well for this condition when it is combined with lipoic acid.[39,40]

Eczema

Despite the fact that GLA (evening primrose oil) is widely used in Europe to treat eczema, the evidence that it works is mixed at best.

A 1989 review of the literature found significant benefit in the nine double-blind controlled studies performed to that date.[41] Evening primrose oil seemed especially effective in relieving itching. However, this review has been sharply criticized for including poorly designed studies and possibly misinterpreting study results.[42]

Improvements in symptoms other than itching were seen in a double-blind study of 48 children with eczema.[43]

However, other research has failed to find any benefit. For example, a 16-week, double-blind study involving 58 children with eczema found no difference between the effects of evening primrose oil and placebo.[44] A 24-week, double-blind study of 160 adults with eczema, who were given either placebo or GLA from borage oil, also found no benefit.[45]

In addition, negative results were seen in a 16-week, double-blind placebo-controlled study of 102 individuals with eczema.[46] Another double-blind trial followed 39 people with hand dermatitis for 24 weeks. Evening primrose oil at a dosage of 6 g daily produced no significant improvement as compared to the placebo.[47]

Rheumatoid Arthritis

According to many studies, fish oil, a source of omega-3 essential fatty acids, definitely improves symptoms of rheumatoid arthritis. A few studies suggest that GLA may also work. One double-blind study followed 56 people with rheumatoid arthritis for 6 months.[48] Participants received either 2.8 g daily of GLA or placebo. The group taking GLA experienced significantly fewer symptoms than the placebo group, and the improvements grew over time.

Other small studies have found similar results.[49,50] The overall conclusion appears to be that purified GLA may offer some benefit for rheumatoid arthritis, especially when used along with standard treatment for rheumatoid arthritis.[51]

Raynaud's Phenomenon

High dosages of evening primrose oil may be useful for Raynaud's phenomenon, a condition in which a person's hands and feet show abnormal sensitivity to cold temperature. A small double-blind study found that GLA produced significantly better results than placebo.[52,53] Similar results have been obtained with the omega-3 fatty acids found in fish oil.

Osteoporosis

Essential fatty acids, when combined with calcium, may also help prevent osteoporosis. In one study, 65 postmenopausal women were given calcium along with either placebo or a combination of omega-6 fatty acids (from evening primrose oil) and omega-3 fatty acids (from fish oil) for a period of 18 months. At the end of the study period, both treated groups had higher bone density and fewer fractures than the placebo group.[54] Similar results were seen in another study of 40 women.[55]

Weight Loss

In a 12-week, double-blind study of 100 obese women, treatment with evening primrose oil failed to produce any weight loss as compared to placebo.[56]

Safety Issues

Most of the safety information we have regarding GLA comes from experience with evening primrose oil.

Animal studies suggest that evening primrose oil is completely nontoxic and noncarcinogenic.[57] Over 4,000 people have taken GLA or evening primrose oil in scientific studies, and no significant adverse effects have ever been noted. However, somewhat less than 2% of the study participants who took evening primrose oil complained of mild headaches and/or gastrointestinal distress, especially at higher dosages.[58,59]

Early reports suggested the possibility that GLA might worsen temporal lobe epilepsy, but there has been no later confirmation.[60]

The maximum safe dosage of GLA for young children, pregnant or nursing women, or those with severe liver or kidney disease has not been established.

GLUCOSAMINE

Supplement Forms/Alternate Names
Glucosamine Hydrochloride, Glucosamine Sulfate, N-Acetyl Glucosamine
Principal Proposed Uses
Osteoarthritis (Relieving Symptoms and Slowing the Course of the Disease)
Other Proposed Uses
Tendinitis, Muscle Injury Prevention

Glucosamine, most commonly used in the form glucosamine sulfate, is a simple molecule derived from glucose, the principal sugar found in blood. In glucosamine, one oxygen atom in glucose is replaced by a nitrogen atom. The chemical term for this modified form of glucose is *amino sugar*.

Glucosamine is produced naturally in the body, where it is a key building block for making cartilage. In Europe, glucosamine is widely used to treat osteoarthritis. Studies show that glucosamine supplements relieve pain and other arthritis symptoms. Interestingly, these improvements seem to last for several weeks after glucosamine supplements are discontinued.

This observation has led to the exciting idea that glucosamine may actually make a deep change in osteoarthritis, rather than simply relieving symptoms. Conventional treatments for arthritis reduce the symptoms but don't slow the actual progress of the disease; in fact, nonsteroidal anti-inflammatory drugs, such as indomethacin, may actually speed the progression of osteoarthritis by interfering with cartilage repair and promoting cartilage destruction.[1-5]

In contrast, glucosamine appears to go beyond treating the symptoms to actually slowing the disease itself. (Chondroitin sulfate and SAMe may do the same.) If this is true, it would represent a revolutionary breakthrough in the treatment of arthritis.

Some athletes use glucosamine, in the (unproved) belief that it can prevent muscle injuries, relieve tendinitis, and repair damaged cartilage.

Sources

There is no U.S. Recommended Dietary Allowance for glucosamine. Your body makes all the glucosamine it needs from building blocks found in foods.

Glucosamine is not usually obtained directly from food. Glucosamine supplements are derived from chitin, a substance found in the shells of shrimp, lobsters, and crabs.

Therapeutic Dosages

For osteoarthritis, a typical dosage of glucosamine is 500 mg 3 times daily. A 1,500-mg dose taken once daily may also be effective.[6] Be patient: results take weeks to develop. Glucosamine is available in three forms: glucosamine sulfate, glucosamine hydrochloride, and N-acetyl glucosamine. All three forms are sold as tablets or capsules. There is some dispute over which form is best.

Glucosamine is often sold in combination with chondroitin. Preliminary information from one animal study suggests that this mixture may be superior to either treatment alone.[7]

Therapeutic Uses

Glucosamine is used to treat osteoarthritis. The research indicates that it is effective, and about equal in strength to low dosages of nonsteroidal anti-inflammatory drugs such as ibuprofen.[8–12] It reduces pain and swelling and improves mobility with results that continue for weeks after treatment stops. It also appears to help prevent progressive joint damage, thereby slowing the course of the disease.[13]

Glucosamine has also been proposed to treat tendinitis, to prevent muscle injuries, and to repair damaged cartilage, but there is as yet no evidence that it is effective.

What Is the Scientific Evidence for Glucosamine for Osteoarthritis?

Symptom Relief

Solid evidence indicates that glucosamine supplements effectively relieve pain and other symptoms of osteoarthritis. Two types of studies have been performed, those that compared glucosamine against placebo and those that compared it against standard medications.

A recent double-blind study compared glucosamine sulfate against placebo in 252 people with osteoarthritis of the knee.[14] After 4 weeks, the group that was given glucosamine experienced significantly reduced pain and improved movement, to a greater extent than the improvements seen in the placebo group.

Another double-blind study followed 329 people who were divided into four groups. One group was given the standard antiarthritis drug piroxicam (Feldene), a second was given glucosamine, a third received both treatments, and the fourth received placebo only.[15,16] Over 90 days, piroxicam and glucosamine proved equally effective at reducing symptoms. Interestingly, the combination treatment (piroxicam plus glucosamine) didn't produce significantly better results than either treatment taken alone.

After 90 days, treatment was stopped and the participants were followed for an additional 60 days. The benefits of piroxicam rapidly disappeared, but the benefits of glucosamine lasted for the full 60 days.

Similar results have been seen in other studies that compared glucosamine against ibuprofen.[17,18]

Slowing the Course of the Disease

A 3-year double-blind placebo-controlled study of 212 individuals found that glucosamine can protect joints from further damage.[19] Over the course of the study, individuals given glucosamine showed some actual improvement in pain and mobility, while those given placebo worsened steadily. Even more importantly, x rays showed that glucosamine treatment prevented progressive damage to the knee joint.

We don't know exactly how glucosamine works. However, besides serving as a basic building block for cartilage, glucosamine appears to stimulate cartilage cells in your joints to make proteoglycans and collagen, two proteins essential for the proper function of joints.[20–24]

Glucosamine may also help prevent collagen from breaking down.[25]

Safety Issues

Glucosamine appears to be extremely safe for people of all ages. No significant side effects have been reported in any of the studies of glucosamine. However, recent case reports and animal studies have raised concerns that glucosamine might be harmful for individuals with diabetes. It may raise blood sugar levels[26–29] and also increase the risk of long-term diabetes side effects such as cataracts.[30]

GLUTAMINE

Supplement Forms/Alternate Names
L-Glutamine

Principal Proposed Uses
There are no well-documented uses for glutamine.

Other Proposed Uses
Post-Exercise Respiratory Infection, Recovery from Critical Illness, Food Allergies

Digestive Disorders: Irritable Bowel Syndrome, Crohn's Disease, Ulcerative Colitis

Overtraining Syndrome, Attention Deficit Disorder, Ulcers, "Brain Booster"

Glutamine, or L-glutamine, is an amino acid derived from another amino acid, glutamic acid. Glutamine plays a role in the health of the immune system, digestive tract, and muscle cells, as well as other bodily functions. It appears to serve as a fuel for the cells that line the intestines. Heavy exercise, infection, surgery, and trauma can deplete the body's glutamine reserves, particularly in muscle cells.

The fact that glutamine does so many good things in the body has led people to try glutamine supplements as a treatment for various conditions, including preventing the infections that often follow endurance exercise, reducing symptoms of overtraining syndrome, improving nutrition in critical illness, alleviating allergies, and treating digestive problems.

Sources

There is no daily requirement for glutamine, because the body can make its own supply. As mentioned earlier, various severe stresses may result in a temporary glutamine deficiency.

High-protein foods such as meat, fish, beans, and dairy products are excellent sources of glutamine.

Therapeutic Dosages

Therapeutic dosages of glutamine range from 1.5 to 6 g daily, divided into several separate doses.

Therapeutic Uses

Endurance athletes frequently catch an infectious illness after completing a marathon or similar forms of exercise. Preliminary evidence suggests that glutamine (like vitamin C) might help prevent such infections.[1,2]

Glutamine (often combined with other nutrients) might be useful as a nutritional supplement for people undergoing recovery from critical illness.[3]

It has also been suggested as a treatment for food allergies, based on a theory called "leaky gut syndrome." This theory holds that in some people whole proteins leak through the wall of the digestive tract and enter the blood, causing allergic reactions. Preliminary evidence suggests that glutamine supplements might reduce leakage through the intestinal walls.[4,5] On the same principle, glutamine supplements have been suggested for people with other digestive problems, such as irritable bowel syndrome, Crohn's disease, ulcerative colitis, and the digestive distress caused by cancer chemotherapy. However, there is no real evidence that it works for these conditions.

Based on glutamine's role in muscle, it has been suggested that glutamine might be useful for athletes experiencing overtraining syndrome. As the name suggests, this syndrome is the cumulative effect of a training regimen that allows too little rest and recovery between workouts. Symptoms include depression, fatigue, reduced performance, and physiological signs of stress. Glutamine supplements have additionally been proposed as treatment for attention deficit disorder, ulcers, and as a "brain booster." However, there is little to no scientific evidence for any of these uses.

What Is the Scientific Evidence for Glutamine?

Infections in Athletes

A double-blind placebo-controlled study evaluated the benefits of supplemental glutamine (5 g) taken at the end of exercise in 151 endurance athletes.[6] The result showed a significant decrease in infections among treated athletes. Only 19% of the athletes taking glutamine got sick, as compared to 51% of those on placebo. Although we don't know how glutamine works to prevent these infections, there is some evidence that it may function by stimulating certain aspects of the immune system.[7]

Recovery from Critical Illness

One small double-blind study found that glutamine supplements might have significant nutritional benefits for seriously ill people.[8] In this study, 84 critically ill hospital patients were divided into two groups. All the patients were being fed through a feeding tube. One group received a normal feeding-tube diet, whereas the other group received this diet plus supplemental glutamine. After 6 months, 14 of the 42 patients receiving glutamine had died, compared with 24 of the control group. The glutamine group also left both the intensive care ward and the hospital significantly sooner than the patients who did not receive glutamine.

Cancer Chemotherapy

A double-blind trial of 65 women undergoing chemotherapy for advanced breast cancer sought to discover whether glutamine at a dose of 30 g per day could reduce chemotherapy-induced diarrhea.[9] The results did not show any benefit from glutamine treatment.

Crohn's Disease

Because glutamine is the major fuel source for cells of the small intestine, glutamine has been proposed as a treatment for Crohn's disease, a disease of the small intestine. However, a double-blind trial of 14 individuals found no benefit.[10]

Safety Issues

As a naturally occurring amino acid, glutamine is thought to
be a safe supplement when taken at recommended dosages.
However, those who are hypersensitive to monosodium glutamate (MSG) should use glutamine with caution, as the
body metabolizes glutamine into glutamate. Also, because
many anti-epilepsy drugs work by blocking glutamate stimu-
lation in the brain, high dosages of glutamine may over-
whelm these drugs and pose a risk to people with epilepsy.

Maximum safe dosages for young children, pregnant or
nursing women, or those with severe liver or kidney disease
have not been determined.

⚠ Interactions You Should Know About

If you are taking **antiseizure medications**, including **carbamazepine**, **phenobarbital**, **Dilantin (phenytoin)**,
Mysoline (primidone), and **valproic acid (Depakene)**,
use glutamine only under medical supervision.

HISTIDINE

Supplement Forms/Alternate Names
L-Histidine
Principal Proposed Uses
There are no well-documented uses for histidine.
Other Proposed Uses
Rheumatoid Arthritis

Histidine is a semiessential amino acid, which means your
body normally makes as much as it needs. Like most other
amino acids, histidine is used to make proteins and enzymes.
The body also uses histidine to make histamine, the culprit behind the swelling and itching you feel in an allergic reaction.

It appears that people with rheumatoid arthritis may
have low levels of histidine in their blood. This has led to
some speculation that histidine supplements might be a good

treatment for this kind of arthritis, but so far no studies have confirmed this.

Sources

Although histidine is not required in the diet, histidine deficiencies can occur during periods of very rapid growth. Dairy products, meat, poultry, fish, and other protein-rich foods are good sources of histidine.

Therapeutic Dosages

A typical therapeutic dosage of histidine is 4 to 5 g daily.

Therapeutic Uses

Although individuals with rheumatoid arthritis appear to have reduced levels of histidine in the blood,[1,2] this by itself doesn't prove that taking histidine will help. One study designed to evaluate this question directly found no significant benefit.[3]

Safety Issues

As a necessary nutrient, histidine is believed to be safe. However, maximum safe dosages of histidine have not been determined for young children, pregnant or nursing women, or those with severe liver or kidney disease. As with other supplements taken in large doses, it is important to purchase a quality product, as contaminants present even in very small percentages could conceivably add up and become toxic.

HMB (HYDROXYMETHYL BUTYRATE)

Supplement Forms/Alternate Names
Beta-Hydroxy Beta-Methylbutyric Acid
Principal Proposed Uses
Muscle Building for Strength Athletes and Bodybuilders

Technically "beta-hydroxy beta-methylbutyric acid," HMB is a chemical that occurs naturally in the body when the amino acid leucine breaks down.

Leucine is found in particularly high concentrations in muscles. During athletic training, damage to the muscles leads to the breakdown of leucine as well as increased HMB levels. Based on the laws of chemistry, it is possible that taking extra HMB might work in the reverse way, slowing loss of muscle tissue. For this reason, HMB has been proposed as a sports supplement for strength athletes and bodybuilders. However, there is little real evidence as yet that it is effective.

Sources

HMB is not an essential nutrient, so there is no established requirement. HMB is found in small amounts in citrus fruit and catfish. To get a therapeutic dosage, however, you need to take a supplement in powder or pill form.

Therapeutic Dosages

A typical therapeutic dosage of HMB is 3 to 5 g daily.

Be careful not to confuse HMB with gamma hydroxybutyrate (GHB), a similar supplement. GHB can cause severe sedation, especially when combined with other sedating substances, such as alcohol or antianxiety drugs.

Therapeutic Uses

Studies evaluating whether HMB can help power athletes increase strength and muscle mass have shown contradictory results.[1–4]

What Is the Scientific Evidence for HMB (Hydroxymethyl Butyrate)?

Muscle Building

Studies on chick and rat muscles suggest that HMB reduces the amount of muscle protein that breaks down during exercise.[5]

In a controlled study, 41 male volunteers aged 19 to 29 were given either 0, 1.5, or 3 g of HMB daily for 3 weeks.[6] The participants also lifted weights 3 days a week for 90 minutes. The results suggest that HMB can enhance strength and muscle mass in direct proportion to how much you take.

In another controlled study reported in the same article, 32 male volunteers took either 3 g of HMB daily or placebo, and then lifted weights for 2 or 3 hours daily, 6 days a week for 7 weeks. The HMB group saw a significantly greater increase in its bench-press strength than the placebo group. However, there was no significant difference in body weight or fat mass by the end of the study.

Two placebo-controlled studies in women found that 3 g of HMB had no effect on lean body mass and strength in sedentary women, but HMB did provide an additional benefit when combined with resistance exercise.[7]

However, two double-blind placebo-controlled studies, each lasting 28 days, failed to detect any effect on body composition or strength.[8] The first enrolled 52 college football players during off-season training, and the other followed 40 athletes engaged in weight training. HMB at a dose of 3 or 6 g daily produced no effect different from placebo.

All of these studies were small, and therefore, their results are not reliable. Larger studies will be necessary to truly establish whether HMB is effective.

Safety Issues

HMB seems to be safe when taken at standard doses.[9] However, full safety studies have not been performed, so HMB should not be used by young children, pregnant or nursing women, or those with severe liver or kidney disease, except on the advice of a physician.

As with all supplements taken in very large doses, it is important to purchase a quality product, as an impurity present even in very small percentages could add up to a real problem.

HUPERZINE A

Principal Proposed Uses
Alzheimer's Disease, Other Forms of Dementia, Ordinary Age-Related Memory Loss

Huperzine A (HUP-er-zeen) is an extremely potent chemical derived from a particular type of club moss (*Huperzia serrata* [Thumb] Trev.). Like caffeine and cocaine, huperzine A is a medicinally active, plant-derived chemical that belongs to the class known as alkaloids. It was first isolated in 1948 by Chinese scientists.[1] This substance is really more a drug than an herb, but it is sold over the counter as a dietary supplement for memory loss and mental impairment.

What Is the Scientific Evidence for Huperzine A?

Many experiments have found that huperzine A can improve memory skills in aged animals as well as in younger animals whose memories have been deliberately impaired.[2–17]

Some of the best research on humans so far was done in a clinical trial involving 103 people with Alzheimer's disease. Participants in this placebo-controlled study were given either huperzine A or placebo twice a day for 8 weeks. About 60% of the treated participants showed improvements in memory, thinking, and behavioral functions compared to 36% of the placebo-treated group. No severe side effects were reported, and the authors concluded that huperzine A is a promising drug for symptomatic treatment of Alzheimer's disease.[18]

Huperzine A inhibits the enzyme acetylcholinesterase (uh-SEE-tul-co-lin-ES-ter-ase). This enzyme breaks down acetylcholine, which seems to play an important role in mental function. When the enzyme that breaks it down is inhibited, acetylcholine levels in the brain tend to rise. Drugs that inhibit acetylcholinesterase (such as tacrine and donepezil) seem to improve memory and mental functioning in people with Alzheimer's and other severe conditions. The research on huperzine A indicates that it works in much the same way.

The chemical action of huperzine A is very precise and specific. It "fits" into a niche on the enzyme where acetylcholine is supposed to attach.[19,20] Because huperzine A is in the way, the enzyme can't grab and destroy acetylcholine. This mechanism has been demonstrated by considerable scientific work, including sophisticated computer modeling of the shape of the molecule.[21]

Although it originally comes from a plant, huperzine A is highly purified in a laboratory and is just a single chemical. It is just not much like an herb. Herbs contain hundreds or thousands of chemicals. In this way, huperzine A resembles drugs such as digoxin, codeine, Sudafed, and vincristine (a chemotherapy drug), which are also highly purified chemicals taken from plants. If we wish to call huperzine A a natural treatment, we need to call these (and dozens of other standard drugs) natural as well.

Dosage

Huperzine A is a highly potent compound with a recommended dose of only 100 to 200 mcg twice daily for age-related memory loss. We recommend using it only under a doctor's supervision.

Safety Issues

Perhaps because it works so specifically, huperzine A appears to have few side effects. However, children, pregnant or nursing women, or those with high blood pressure or severe liver or kidney disease should not take huperzine A except on a doctor's recommendation. We also don't know whether huperzine A interacts adversely with any drugs.

HYDROXYCITRIC ACID

Supplement Forms/Alternate Names
Garcinia cambogia, Gorikapuli, HCA, Hydroxycitrate, Malabar Tamarind
Principal Proposed Uses
There are no well-documented uses for hydroxycitric acid.
Other Proposed Uses
Weight Loss

Hydroxycitric acid (HCA), a derivative of citric acid, is found primarily in a small, sweet, purple fruit called the Malabar tamarind or, as it is most commonly called, *Garcinia cambogia.* Test-tube and animal research suggests that HCA may be helpful in weight loss because of its effects on metabolism. However, a recent, well-designed study found it ineffective.

Sources

HCA is not an essential nutrient. The Malabar tamarind is the only practical source of this supplement.

Therapeutic Dosages

A typical dosage of HCA is 250 to 1,000 mg 3 times daily. Supplements are available in many forms, including tablets, capsules, powders, and even snack bars. Products are often labeled *Garcinia cambogia* and standardized to contain a fixed percentage of HCA.

Therapeutic Uses

According to animal studies, HCA can suppress appetite and thereby encourage weight loss.[1–5] It is thought to work by interfering with the body's ability to produce and store fat.[6–9] However, the largest and best-designed human trial found no benefit.[10] Another small, placebo-controlled study found no effect on metabolism.[11]

What Is the Scientific Evidence for Hydroxycitric Acid?

A 12-week double-blind placebo-controlled trial of 135 over-weight individuals, who were given either placebo or 500 mg of HCA (as *Garcinia cambogia* extract standardized to contain 50% HCA) three times daily, found no effect on body weight or fat mass.[12] Another study tested HCA to see if it could cause weight loss by affecting metabolism, but no effects on metabolism were found.[13]

Safety Issues

The Malabar tamarind (from which HCA is extracted) is a traditional food and flavoring in Southeast Asia. No serious side effects have been reported from animal or human studies involving either fruit extracts or the concentrated chemical. However, formal safety studies have not been performed, and therefore, its safety remains unknown.

INOSINE

Principal Proposed Uses
There are no well-documented uses for inosine.
Other Proposed Uses
Athletic Performance, Heart Disease, Tourette's Syndrome

Inosine is an important chemical found throughout the body. It plays many roles, one of which is helping to make ATP (adenosine triphosphate), the body's main form of usable energy. Based primarily on this fact, inosine supplements have been proposed as an energy-booster for athletes, as well as a treatment for various heart conditions.

Sources

Inosine is not an essential nutrient. However, brewer's yeast and organ meats, such as liver and kidney, contain considerable amounts. Inosine is also available in purified form.

Therapeutic Dosages

When used as a sports supplement, a typical dosage of inosine is 5 to 6 g daily.

Therapeutic Uses

Inosine has been proposed as a treatment for various forms of heart disease, from inflammation of the heart lining to irregular heartbeat and heart attacks. However, the evidence that it works is highly preliminary.[1]

Inosine is better known as a performance enhancer for athletes, although most of the available evidence suggests that it doesn't work for this purpose.[2–5]

Inosine has also been suggested as a possible treatment for Tourette's syndrome, a neurological disorder.[6]

Safety Issues

Although no side effects have been reported with the use of inosine, comprehensive safety studies have not been completed. For this reason, young children, pregnant or nursing women, or those with serious liver or kidney disease should not use inosine.

As with all supplements taken in multigram doses, it is important to purchase a reputable product, because a contaminant present even in small percentages could add up to a real problem.

INOSITOL

Supplement Forms/Alternate Names
Vitamin B_8
Principal Proposed Uses
Depression, Panic Disorder
Other Proposed Uses
Alzheimer's Disease, Obsessive-Compulsive Disorder, Attention Deficit Disorder, Diabetic Neuropathy

Inositol, unofficially referred to as vitamin B_8, is present in all animal tissues, with the highest levels in the heart and brain. It is part of the membranes (outer linings) of all cells, and plays a role in helping the liver process fats as well as contributing to the function of muscles and nerves.

Inositol may also be involved in depression. People who are depressed have much lower-than-normal levels of inositol in their spinal fluid. In addition, inositol participates in the action of *serotonin,* a neurotransmitter known to be a factor in depression. (Neurotransmitters are chemicals that transmit messages between nerve cells.) For this reason, inositol has been proposed as a treatment for depression, and preliminary evidence suggests that it may be helpful.

Inositol has also been tried for other psychological and nerve-related conditions.

Sources

Inositol is not known to be an essential nutrient. However, nuts, seeds, beans, whole grains, cantaloupe, and citrus fruits supply a substance called phytic acid, which releases inositol when acted on by bacteria in the digestive tract. The typical American diet provides an estimated 1,000 mg daily.

Therapeutic Dosages

Experimentally, inositol dosages of up to 18 g daily have been tried for various conditions.

Therapeutic Uses

Preliminary double-blind studies suggest that high-dose inositol may be useful for depression,[1,2,3] panic disorder,[4] Alzheimer's disease,[5] obsessive-compulsive disorder,[6] and attention deficit disorder.[7]

Inositol is also sometimes proposed as a treatment for complications of diabetes, specifically diabetic neuropathy, but there have been no double-blind placebo-controlled studies, and two uncontrolled studies had mixed results.[8,9]

What Is the Scientific Evidence for Inositol?

Depression

Small double-blind studies have found inositol helpful for depression.[10,11] In one such trial, 28 depressed individuals were given a daily dose of 12 g of inositol for 4 weeks.[12] By the fourth week, the group receiving inositol showed significant improvement compared to the placebo group. However, by itself this study was too small to prove anything.

Panic Disorder

People with panic disorder frequently develop panic attacks, often with no warning. The racing heartbeat, chest pressure, sweating, and other physical symptoms can be so intense that they are mistaken for a heart attack. A small double-blind study (21 participants) found that people given 12 g of inositol daily had fewer, and less severe, panic attacks as compared to the placebo group.[13] Again, this study was too small to prove anything.

Safety Issues

No serious ill effects have been reported for inositol, even with a therapeutic dosage that equals about 18 times the average dietary intake. However, no long-term safety studies have been performed. Safety has not been established in young children, women who are pregnant or nursing, and those with severe liver and kidney disease. As with all supplements used in multigram doses, it is important to purchase a reputable product, because a contaminant present even in small percentages could add up to a real problem.

IODINE

Supplement Forms/Alternate Names
Elemental Iodine, Iodide

Principal Proposed Uses
Correcting Nutritional Deficiency

Other Proposed Uses
Cyclic Mastalgia

Your thyroid gland, located just above the middle of your collarbone, needs iodine to make thyroid hormone, which maintains normal metabolism in all cells of the body. Principally found in sea water, dietary iodine can be scarce in many inland areas, and deficiencies were common before iodine was added to table salt. Iodine deficiency causes enlargement of the thyroid, a condition known as goiter. However, if you are not deficient in iodine, taking extra iodine will not help your thyroid work better, and it might even cause problems.

For reasons that are not clear, supplementary iodine might also be helpful for cyclic mastalgia.

Requirements/Sources

The U.S. Recommended Dietary Allowance for iodine is

- Infants under 6 months, 40 mcg
  6 to 12 months, 50 mcg
- Children 1 to 3 years, 70 mcg
  4 to 6 years, 90 mcg
  7 to 10 years, 120 mcg
- Adults (and children 11 years and older), 150 mcg
- Pregnant women, 175 mcg
- Nursing women, 200 mcg

Iodine deficiency is rare in developed countries today because of the use of iodized salt.

Seafood and kelp contain very high levels of iodine, as do salty processed foods that use iodized salt.

Most iodine is in the form of iodide, but a few studies suggest that a special form of iodine called molecular iodine may be better than iodide (see What Is the Scientific Evidence for Iodine?).

Therapeutic Dosages

A typical therapeutic dosage of iodide or iodine is 200 mcg daily.

Therapeutic Uses

Iodine supplements have been proposed as a treatment for cyclic mastalgia (breast pain and lumpiness that usually cycles in relation to the menstrual period, also called cyclic mastitis or fibrocystic breast disease).[1]

What Is the Scientific Evidence for Iodine?

Cyclic Mastalgia (Cyclic Mastitis, Fibrocystic Breast Disease)

Three clinical studies indicate that supplements providing iodine may be helpful in treating cyclic mastalgia.[2] These studies suggest that either iodide or iodine (the pure molecular form) might be useful. In the one placebo-controlled trial among this group, a study that enrolled 56 individuals, molecular iodine was found superior to placebo in relieving pain and reducing the number of cysts.

Another of these studies compared molecular iodine to iodide. Molecular iodine was no more effective than iodide, but was deemed superior because it induced fewer side effects and did not affect the thyroid.

Safety Issues

When taken at the recommended dosage, iodine and iodide appear to be safe nutritional supplements. However, excessive doses of iodide can actually cause thyroid problems! There is also a speculative link between excessive iodide intake and thyroid cancer. For these reasons, iodide intake above about 200 mcg daily is not recommended.

IPRIFLAVONE

Principal Proposed Uses
Preventing and Treating Osteoporosis
Other Proposed Uses
Reducing the Pain of Osteoporotic Fractures, Bodybuilding

Isoflavones are water-soluble chemicals found in many plants. Ipriflavone is a semisynthetic version of an isoflavone found in soy.

Soy isoflavones have effects in the body somewhat similar to those of estrogen. This should be beneficial, but it is possible that soy could present some of the risks of estrogen as well. In 1969, a research project was initiated to manufacture a type of isoflavone that would possess the bone-stimulating effects of estrogen without any estrogen-like activity elsewhere in the body. Such a product would help prevent osteoporosis but cause no other health risks.

Ipriflavone was the result. After 7 successful years of experiments with animals, human research was started in 1981. Today, ipriflavone is available in over 22 countries and in most drugstores in the United States as a nonprescription dietary supplement. It is an accepted treatment for osteoporosis in Italy, Turkey, and Japan.

Like estrogen, ipriflavone appears to slow and perhaps slightly reverse bone breakdown. It also seems to help reduce the pain of fractures caused by osteoporosis. However, since it does not appear to have any estrogenic effects anywhere else in the body, it shouldn't increase the risk of breast or uterine cancer. On the other hand, it won't reduce the hot flashes, night sweats, mood changes, or vaginal dryness of menopause, nor prevent heart disease. Ipriflavone is also touted as a bodybuilding aid, but no real evidence supports this use.

Sources

Ipriflavone is not an essential nutrient and is not found to any appreciable extent in food. It must be taken as a supplement.

Therapeutic Dosages

The proper dosage of ipriflavone is 200 mg 3 times daily, or 300 mg twice daily.

Therapeutic Uses

Ipriflavone appears to be able to slow down and perhaps slightly reverse osteoporosis. It may be helpful for this purpose in ordinary postmenopausal osteoporosis as well as osteoporosis caused by medications.[1–17] Ipriflavone also seems to ease the pain of fractures caused by osteoporosis.[18,19,20] There is no real evidence that it is helpful for bodybuilding.

What Is the Scientific Evidence for Ipriflavone?

Preventing and Treating Osteoporosis

Numerous double-blind placebo-controlled studies involving a total of over 1,000 participants have examined the effects of ipriflavone on osteoporosis.[21–25] Overall, it appears that ipriflavone can slow the progression of osteoporosis and perhaps reverse it to some extent. For example, a 2-year double-blind study followed 198 postmenopausal women who showed evidence of bone loss.[26] At the end of the study, there was a gain in bone density of 1% in the ipriflavone group and a loss of 0.7% in the placebo group. These numbers may sound small, but they can add up to a lot of bone over time.

Ipriflavone, like estrogen, probably works by fighting bone breakdown.[27–30] However, there is some evidence that it may also increase new bone formation, too.[31–33]

In Combination with Calcium

Taking calcium plus ipriflavone may also be an excellent idea. In one study, 60 women who had already been diagnosed with osteoporosis and had already suffered one spinal fracture were given either 1,000 mg of calcium or 1,000 mg of calcium with ipriflavone.[34] After 6 months, the ipriflavone group had an increase of bone density in the spine of 3.5%, compared to a net loss in the calcium-only group.

In Combination with Estrogen

Combining ipriflavone with estrogen may enhance anti-osteoporosis benefits.[35,36] However, we do not know for sure whether such combinations increase or reduce the other risks (or benefits) of estrogen (see Safety Issues).

Preventing Side Effects of Medications

Ipriflavone may also be helpful for preventing osteoporosis in women who are taking Lupron or corticosteroids, medications that accelerate bone loss.[37,38]

Reducing Pain of Fractures Caused by Osteoporosis

For reasons that are not at all clear, ipriflavone appears to be able to reduce pain in osteoporosis-related fractures that have already occurred.[39,40,41]

Safety Issues

Nearly 3,000 people have used ipriflavone in clinical studies, with no more side effects than those taking placebo.[42] However, one study suggests that ipriflavone might sometimes reduce white blood cell count; therefore, it should not be used by anyone with immune deficiencies. Because ipriflavone is metabolized by the kidneys, individuals with severe kidney disease should have their ipriflavone dosage monitored by a physician.[43]

Also, although ipriflavone itself does not affect tissues outside of bone, some evidence suggests that if it is combined with estrogen, estrogen's effects on the uterus are increased.[44,45] This might mean that the risk of uterine cancer would be elevated over taking estrogen alone. It should be possible to overcome this risk by taking progesterone along with estrogen, which is standard medical practice in any case. However, this finding does make one wonder whether ipriflavone–estrogen combinations raise the risk of breast cancer too, an estrogen side effect that has no easy solution. At present, there is no available information on this important subject.

Additionally, ipriflavone may interfere with certain drugs by affecting the way they are processed in the liver. For example, it may raise blood levels of the older asthma drug theophylline.[46,47,48] It could also raise levels of caffeine, meaning that if you drink coffee while taking ipriflavone you might stay up longer than you expect! Additionally, ipriflavone could interact with tolbutamide (a drug for diabetes), phenytoin (used for epilepsy), and Coumadin (a blood thinner).[49] Such interactions are potentially dangerous, especially since phenytoin and warfarin cause osteoporosis, and some people might be tempted to try taking ipriflavone at the same time.

⚠ Interactions You Should Know About

If you are taking

- **Theophylline**, **tolbutamide**, **Dilantin (phenytoin)**, **Coumadin (warfarin)**, or any other drug metabolized in the liver: Ipriflavone might change the levels of that drug in your body.
- **Estrogen:** Ipriflavone might help it strengthen your bones even more. However, it might also increase the risk of uterine cancer.

IRON

Supplement Forms/Alternate Names
Chelated Iron, Iron Sulfate

Principal Proposed Uses
Iron Deficiency Anemia

Other Proposed Uses
Menorrhagia (Heavy Menstruation), Attention Deficit Disorder

The element iron is essential to human life. As part of hemoglobin, the oxygen-carrying protein found in red blood cells, iron plays an integral role in nourishing every cell in the body with oxygen. It also functions as a part of myoglobin, which helps muscle cells store oxygen. Without iron, your body could not make ATP (adenosine triphosphate, the body's primary energy source), produce DNA, or carry out many other critical processes.

Iron deficiency can lead to anemia, learning disabilities, impaired immune function, fatigue, and depression. However, you shouldn't take iron supplements unless lab tests show that you are genuinely deficient.

There are two major forms of iron: heme iron and nonheme iron. Heme iron is bound to the proteins hemoglobin or myoglobin, whereas nonheme iron is an inorganic compound. (In chemistry, "organic" has a very precise meaning that has nothing to do with farming. An organic compound contains carbon atoms. Thus "inorganic iron" is an iron compound containing no carbon.) Heme iron, obtained from red meats and fish, is easily absorbed by the body. Nonheme iron, derived from plants, is less easily absorbed.

Requirements/Sources

The U.S. Recommended Dietary Allowance is as follows

- Infants under 6 months, 6 mg
- Children 6 months to 10 years, 10 mg
- Males 11 to 18 years, 12 mg
    19 years and older, 10 mg
- Females 11 to 50 years, 15 mg
    51 years and older, 10 mg
- Menstruating women, 15 mg
- Pregnant women, 30 mg
- Nursing women, 15 mg

Iron deficiency is the most common nutrient deficiency in the world[1] and the number-one cause of anemia. In developed countries, deficiency is much more common in menstruating women than in men. Other groups at high risk are children and pregnant women.[2]

Rich sources of heme iron include oysters, meat, poultry, and fish. The main sources of nonheme iron are dried fruits, molasses, whole grains, legumes, egg yolks, leafy green vegetables, nuts, seeds, and kelp. Acidic foods, such as fruit preserves and tomatoes, are a good source of iron when they've been cooked in iron or stainless steel cookware (some of the iron leaches into the food).

Iron can interfere with the absorption of numerous medications, including captopril, levodopa, carbidopa, penicillamine, thyroid hormone, and antibiotics in the tetracycline or quinolone (Floxin, Cipro) family.[3]

Therapeutic Dosages

The typical short-term therapeutic dosage to correct iron deficiency is 100 to 200 mg daily. Once your body's iron stores reach normal levels, however, this dose should be reduced to the lowest level that can maintain iron balance.

Therapeutic Uses

The most obvious use of iron supplements is to treat iron deficiency anemia. However, don't take iron just because you feel tired. Make sure to get tested to see whether you are indeed deficient. With iron, more is definitely not better.

Heavy menstruation (menorrhagia) can certainly cause iron loss. However, for reasons that are not clear, iron supplementation can reportedly lighten up heavy menstrual bleeding, but only if you are iron deficient to begin with.[4] Iron has also been tried as a treatment for attention deficit disorder, but there is as yet no real evidence that it works.

What Is the Scientific Evidence for Iron?

Menorrhagia

One small double-blind study found good results using iron supplements to treat heavy menstruation. This study, which was performed in 1964, saw an improvement in 75% of the women who took iron (compared to 32.5% of those who took placebo). Women who began with higher iron levels did not respond to treatment.[5] This suggests once more that supplementing with iron is only a good idea if you are deficient in it.

Safety Issues

At the recommended dosage, iron is quite safe. Excessive dosages, however, can be toxic—damaging the intestines and liver, and possibly resulting in death. Iron poisoning in children is a surprisingly common problem, so make sure to keep your iron supplements out of their reach.

Mildly excessive levels of iron may be unhealthy for another reason: it acts as an oxidant (the opposite of an antioxidant), perhaps increasing the risk of cancer and heart disease. Elevated levels of iron may also play a role in brain injury caused by stroke, and might increase complications of pregnancy.

⚠ Interactions You Should Know About

If you are taking

- Antibiotics in the **tetracycline** or **quinolone** (Floxin, Cipro) families, **ACE inhibitors**, **levodopa**, **methyldopa**, **carbidopa**, **penicillamine**, **thyroid hormone**, **calcium**, **soy**,[6] **zinc**,[7] **copper**,[8] or **manganese**[9]: Take iron supplements at a different time of day to avoid absorption problems.
- Drugs that reduce stomach acid such as **H$_2$ blockers** and **proton pump inhibitors**: You may need extra iron.
- High doses of **vitamin C:** You may absorb too much iron.

ISOFLAVONES

Supplement Forms/Alternate Names
Soy Isoflavones, Red Clover Isoflavones
Principal Proposed Uses
High Cholesterol, Menopausal Symptoms
Other Proposed Uses
Osteoporosis, Cancer Prevention

Isoflavones are water-soluble chemicals found in many plants. In this chapter, we will discuss a group of isoflavones that are phytoestrogens, meaning that they cause effects in the body somewhat similar to those of estrogen. The most investigated phytoestrogen isoflavones, genistein and daidzein, are found in soy products and the herb red clover.

One of the ways these isoflavones appear to work is interesting. Although they are less powerful than the body's own estrogen, they latch on to the same places (receptor sites) on cells and don't allow actual estrogen to attach. In this way, when there is not enough estrogen in the body, isoflavones can partially make up for it; but when there is plenty of estrogen, they can partially block its influence. The net effect may be to reduce some of the risks of excess estrogen (breast and uterine cancer) while still providing some of estrogen's benefits (preventing osteoporosis). These isoflavones may work in other ways as well, such as by lowering the body's own level of estrogen.[1,2]

Sources

Although isoflavones are not essential nutrients, they may help reduce the incidence of several diseases. Thus isoflavones may be useful for optimum health, even if they are not necessary for life like a classic vitamin.

Roasted soybeans have the highest isoflavone content: about 167 mg for a 3.5-ounce serving. Tempeh is next, with 60 mg, followed by soy flour with 44 mg. Processed soy products such as soy protein and soy milk contain about 20 mg per serving. The same isoflavones found in soy are also contained in certain red clover products; check the label to determine the content.

Therapeutic Dosages

The optimum dosage of isoflavones obtained from food is not known.

We know that Japanese women eat up to 200 mg of isoflavones from soy daily, but we don't really know what amount of natural isoflavones is ideal. According to one study, 62 mg of isoflavones daily is sufficient to reduce cholesterol.[3]

Therapeutic Uses

Soy products are known to reduce cholesterol, and soy isoflavones appear to be their active ingredient for this purpose.[4,5] Soy isoflavones may also help prevent some forms of cancer.[6–12]

Soy has also been found to reduce menopausal symptoms.[13,14] Although similar results have been expected from red clover isoflavones, studies on their use for menopausal symptoms have not produced positive results.[15,16]

Promising evidence suggests that soy isoflavones may be helpful for preventing osteoporosis.[17–25] However, there is much more evidence for the semisynthetic isoflavone, ipriflavone, for this purpose.

What *don't* soy isoflavones do? They don't seem to lower blood pressure.[26]

What Is the Scientific Evidence for Isoflavones?

High Cholesterol

In 1995, a review of 38 controlled studies on soy and heart disease concluded that soy is definitely effective at reducing total cholesterol, LDL ("bad") cholesterol, and triglycerides.[27] It appears that the isoflavones in soy are the active ingredient.[28]

One double-blind study (not part of the review mentioned previously), which involved 66 older women, found improvements in HDL ("good") cholesterol as well.[29] The women were divided into three groups. The first group received 40 g of skim milk protein daily. The second group was given the same amount of soy protein, and the third received 40 g of soy protein with extra soy isoflavones. Compared with the skim milk (placebo) group, both soy groups showed significant improvements in both total cholesterol and HDL cholesterol.

Menopausal Symptoms ("Hot Flashes")

Soy protein, presumably due to its isoflavone content, seems to relieve "hot flashes," a common symptom of menopause. A double-blind placebo-controlled study involving 104 women found that soy protein provided significant relief compared to placebo (milk protein). After 3 weeks, the women taking daily doses of 60 g of soy protein were having 26% fewer hot flashes.[30] By week 12, the reduction was 45%. Women taking placebo also experienced a big improvement by week 12 (30% fewer hot flashes), but soy gave significantly better results.

However, isoflavones from red clover have not done well in studies on menopausal symptoms. A 28-week, double-blind placebo-controlled crossover trial of 51 postmenopausal women found no reduction in hot flashes among those given 40 mg of red clover isoflavones daily.[31] No benefits were seen in another double-blind placebo-controlled trial, which involved 37 women also given isoflavones from red clover at a dose of either 40 mg or 160 mg daily.[32]

There are many potential explanations for this discrepancy. It may be that the exact mixture of isoflavones in red clover is significantly different from that which is found in soy. Another possibility is that as yet unidentified soy constituents play a role.

Osteoporosis

In one study that evaluated the benefits of soy isoflavones in osteoporosis, a total of 66 postmenopausal women took either placebo (soy protein with isoflavones removed) or 56 or 90 mg of soy isoflavones daily for 6 months.[33] The group that took the higher dosage of isoflavones showed significant gains in spinal bone density. There was little change in the placebo or low-dose isoflavone groups. This study suggests that soy isoflavones may be effective for osteoporosis.

Very nearly the same results were also seen in a similar study. This 24-week, double-blind trial of 69 postmenopausal women found that soy isoflavones can significantly reduce bone loss from the spine.[34]

Similar benefits have been seen in animal studies.[35–41] However, a couple of studies have not found benefit.[42,43]

Estrogen and most other medications for osteoporosis work by fighting bone breakdown. Soy isoflavones may work in the other way, by helping to increase new bone formation.[44,45]

Safety Issues

Natural soy isoflavones have not been subjected to rigorous safety studies. However, because they are consumed in very high quantities among those who eat traditional Asian diets, they are thought to be reasonably safe. Nonetheless, because isoflavones work somewhat like estrogen, there are at least theoretical concerns that they may not be safe for women who have already had breast cancer. Furthermore, evidence from one highly preliminary study in humans found changes suggestive of increased breast cancer risk after women took a commercial soy protein product.[46] Preliminary studies and reports have raised concerns that intensive use of soy products by pregnant women could exert a hormonal effect that impacts unborn fetuses.[47,48]

Red clover isoflavones probably present similar risks.

In addition, soy products may impair thyroid function or reduce absorption of thyroid medication, at least in children.[49,50,51] For this reason, individuals with impaired thyroid function should use soy with caution.

LECITHIN

Supplement Forms/Alternate Names
Egg Lecithin, Phosphatidylcholine in Lecithin, Soy Lecithin

Principal Proposed Uses
There are no well-documented uses for lecithin.

Other Proposed Uses
High Cholesterol, Liver Disease
Psychological and Neurological Disorders: Alzheimer's Disease, Bipolar Disorder, Tourette's Syndrome

For decades, lecithin has been a popular treatment for high cholesterol (although there is surprisingly little evidence that it works). More recently, lecithin has been proposed as a remedy for various psychological and neurological diseases, such as Tourette's syndrome, Alzheimer's disease, and bipolar disorder (also known as manic depression). Lecithin contains a substance called *phosphatidylcholine* (PC) that is presumed to be responsible for its medicinal effects. Phosphatidylcholine is a major part of the membranes surrounding our cells. However, when you consume phosphatidylcholine it is broken down into the nutrient *choline* rather than being carried directly to cell membranes. Choline acts like folate, TMG (trimethylglycine), and SAMe (S-adenosylmethionine) to promote methylation (see the chapter on TMG for further discussion of this subject). It is also used to make *acetylcholine*, a nerve chemical essential for proper brain function.

Sources

Neither lecithin nor its ingredient phosphatidylcholine is an essential nutrient. For use as a supplement or a food additive, lecithin is often manufactured from soy.

Therapeutic Dosages

Ordinary lecithin contains about 10 to 20% phosphatidylcholine. However, European research has tended to use products concentrated to contain 90% phosphatidylcholine in lecithin, and the following dosages are based on that type of product. For psychological and neurological conditions, doses as high as 5 to 10 g taken 3 times daily have been used in studies. For liver disease, a typical dose is 350 to 500 mg taken 3 times daily; and for high cholesterol, 500 to 900 mg taken 3 times daily is common.

Therapeutic Uses

For a while, lecithin/phosphatidylcholine was one of the most commonly recommended natural treatments for high cholesterol. This idea, however, appears to rest entirely on preliminary studies that lacked control groups.[1,2] A recent small, double-blind study of 23 men with high blood cholesterol levels found that lecithin had *no* significant effects on blood levels of total cholesterol, HDL ("good") cholesterol, LDL ("bad") cholesterol, or lipoprotein(a) and triglycerides (two harmful fats found in the blood).[3]

In Europe, phosphatidylcholine is also used to treat liver diseases, such as alcoholic fatty liver and viral hepatitis. While there is some evidence from animal and human studies that it may be helpful, other studies found no benefit.[4–12]

Finally, because phosphatidylcholine plays a role in nerve function, it has also been suggested as a treatment for various psychological and neurological disorders, such as Alzheimer's disease, bipolar disorder, Tourette's syndrome, and tardive dyskinesia (a late-developing side effect of drugs used for psychosis). However, the evidence that it works is limited to small studies with somewhat conflicting results.[13–20]

Safety Issues

Lecithin is believed to be generally safe. However, some people taking high dosages (several grams daily) experience minor but annoying side effects, such as abdominal discomfort, diarrhea, and nausea. Maximum safe dosages for young children, pregnant or nursing women, or those with severe liver or kidney disease have not been determined.

LIPOIC ACID

Supplement Forms/Alternate Names
Alpha-Lipoic Acid, Thioctic Acid
Principal Proposed Uses
Diabetic Peripheral Neuropathy, Diabetic Autonomic Neuropathy
Other Proposed Uses
Diabetes (in General), Liver Disease, Cancer Prevention, Cataract Prevention, Heart Disease Prevention

Lipoic acid, also known as alpha-lipoic acid, is a sulfur-containing fatty acid that has recently become very popular as a dietary supplement. It is found inside every cell of the body, where it helps generate the energy that keeps us alive and functioning. Lipoic acid is a key part of the metabolic machinery that turns glucose (blood sugar) into energy for the body's needs.

Lipoic acid is an antioxidant, which means it neutralizes naturally occurring, but harmful, chemicals known as free radicals. Unlike other antioxidants, which work only in water or fatty tissues, lipoic acid is unusual in that it functions in both water and fat.[1,2] By comparison, vitamin E works only in fat and vitamin C works only in water. This gives lipoic acid an unusually broad spectrum of action.

Different antioxidants work together to keep free radicals under control (for more information, see the chapter on vitamin E). Antioxidants are a bit like kamikaze pilots, sacrificing themselves to knock out free radicals. One of the more interesting findings about lipoic acid is that it may help regenerate other antioxidants that have been used up. Some research also suggests that lipoic acid may do the work of other antioxidants in which the body is deficient.[3,4]

Thanks to its fat solubility, lipoic acid can get inside nerve cells, where it helps prevent free radical damage.

Sources

Because a healthy body makes enough lipoic acid to supply its energy requirements, there is no daily requirement for this supplement. However, several medical conditions appear to be accompanied by low levels of lipoic acid[5]—specifically, diabetes, liver cirrhosis, and heart disease—which suggests (but definitely does not prove) that supplementation would be helpful.

Liver and yeast contain some lipoic acid. Nonetheless, supplements are necessary to obtain therapeutic dosages.

Therapeutic Dosages

The typical dosage of oral lipoic acid for treating complications of diabetes is 300 to 600 mg daily, although much higher doses have been tried in studies. Be patient, as the results take weeks to develop. For use as a general antioxidant, a lower dosage of 20 to 50 mg daily is commonly recommended.

Therapeutic Uses

Lipoic acid has been widely used for decades in Germany to treat diabetic peripheral neuropathy. This is a condition caused by diabetes in which nerves leading to the arms and legs become damaged, leading to numbness, pain, and other symptoms. However, the evidence that it works is largely limited to studies that used the intravenous form of this supplement.[6,7,8]

Lipoic acid has shown promise for another type of nerve damage caused by diabetes: autonomic neuropathy. This is a condition in which the nerves that control internal organs become damaged. When this occurs in the heart, the condition is called cardiac autonomic neuropathy, and it leads to irregularities of heart rhythm. There is some evidence that lipoic acid may be helpful for this condition.[9] When autonomic neuropathy occurs in the intestines, it causes extreme constipation. Based on its other effects, it appears possible that lipoic acid could help this condition as well, although there is no direct evidence to turn to.

Preliminary and sometimes contradictory evidence suggests that lipoic acid may improve other aspects of diabetes as well, including circulation in small blood vessels, metabolism of sugar and protein, and the body's response to insulin.[10-14] Lipoic acid has been proposed as a treatment for liver conditions as well as for preventing cancer, cataracts, and heart disease. However, there is little to no real evidence that it is effective for these purposes.

What Is the Scientific Evidence for Lipoic Acid?

Diabetic Peripheral Neuropathy

There is some evidence that intravenous lipoic acid can reduce symptoms of diabetic peripheral neuropathy, at least in the short term. Oral lipoic acid has not been well evaluated, and the best study of oral lipoic acid found it ineffective for long-term use.

A randomized, double-blind, placebo-controlled study that enrolled 503 individuals with diabetic neuropathy found that intravenous lipoic acid helped reduce symptoms over a 3-week period, but long-term oral supplementation was not effective.[15]

A previous double-blind placebo-controlled study also found short-term benefit with intravenous lipoic acid.[16,17]

Warning: You should never attempt to take any drug or supplement intravenously except under the care of a doctor.

The positive evidence for oral lipoic acid is limited to open studies or to trials that were too small upon which to base conclusions.[18-21]

There is some preliminary evidence that lipoic acid may be more effective if it is combined with GLA (gamma-linolenic acid), another supplement used for diabetic peripheral neuropathy.[22,23]

Diabetic Autonomic Neuropathy

Not only does diabetes damage the nerves in the arms and legs, but it can also affect deep nerves that control organs such as the heart and digestive tract. The DEKAN (Deutsche Kardiale Autonome Neuropathie) study followed 73 people with diabetes who had symptoms caused by nerve damage affecting the heart. Treatment with 800 mg daily of oral lipoic acid showed statistically significant improvement compared to placebo and caused no significant side effects.[24]

Safety Issues

Lipoic acid appears to have no significant side effects at dosages up to 1,800 mg daily.[25] In particular, it does not appear to significantly affect blood sugar levels.

Safety for young children, women who are pregnant or nursing, or those with severe liver or kidney disease has not been established.

LUTEIN

Principal Proposed Uses
There are no well-documented uses for lutein.

Other Proposed Uses
Macular Degeneration, Cataracts, Atherosclerosis

Lutein, a chemical found in green vegetables, is a member of a family of substances known as *carotenoids*. Beta-carotene is the most famous nutrient in this class (for more information, see the chapter on beta carotene). Like beta-carotene, lutein is an antioxidant that protects our cells against damage caused by dangerous, naturally occurring chemicals known as free radicals.

Recent evidence has found that lutein may play an important role in protecting our eyes and eyesight. It may work in two ways: by acting directly as a kind of natural sunblock, and also by neutralizing free radicals that can damage the eye.

Sources

Lutein is not an essential nutrient. However, it may be very important for optimal health. We're learning more all the time about nutrients like lutein that aren't required for life, but protect us in various ways. At present, an intake of about 6 mg daily of lutein is considered adequate.

Green vegetables are the best source of lutein, especially spinach, kale, collard greens, romaine lettuce, leeks, and peas. Unlike beta-carotene, lutein is not found in high concentrations in yellow and orange vegetables such as carrots.

Therapeutic Dosages

We don't know how much lutein is necessary for a therapeutic effect, but estimates range from 5 to 30 mg daily.

Therapeutic Uses

Evidence suggests that people who eat foods containing lutein are less likely to develop macular degeneration or cataracts, the two most common causes of vision loss in adults.[1–4] However, these were observational studies, in which people simply eat what they please and researchers follow them to see what illnesses they develop. Because lutein is found in vegetables that may also contain other helpful substances, we don't know for sure if it is the lutein itself that is providing the benefit. We really need studies in which some people are given pure lutein and others placebo, but as yet they have not been performed.

However, there are reasons to believe that lutein may indeed play an important role in protecting the eyes. Lutein is the main pigment (coloring chemical) in the center of the retina, the region of maximum visual sensitivity known as the macula. Macular degeneration consists of injury to the macula and leads to a severe loss in vision.

One of the main causes of macular degeneration appears to be sun damage to the sensitive tissue. Lutein appears to act as a natural eyeshade, protecting the retina against too much light.[5,6] This may explain why higher dietary intake of lutein appears to reduce the risk of this common cause of blindness in adults.

Besides protecting the macula, lutein may also shield the lens of the eye from light damage, slowing down the development of cataracts.

Furthermore, lutein fights free radicals. These chemicals can also damage the retina and the lens.

Note: Lutein may help prevent macular degeneration, but it has not been proven to treat the condition once it has developed. If you already have macular degeneration, medical supervision is essential.

Lutein might also help prevent atherosclerosis.[7]

Safety Issues

Although lutein is a normal part of the diet, there has not been a formal evaluation of lutein's safety when taken as a concentrated supplement. Maximum safe dosages for young children, pregnant or nursing women, or those with severe liver or kidney disease have not been established.

LYCOPENE

Principal Proposed Uses
Cancer Prevention

Other Proposed Uses
Cataract Prevention, Macular Degeneration Prevention

Lycopene is a powerful antioxidant found in tomatoes, watermelon, guava, and pink grapefruit. Like the better-known supplement beta-carotene, lycopene belongs to the family of chemicals known as *carotenoids* (for more information about carotenoids, see the chapter on beta-carotene). As an antioxidant, it is about twice as powerful as beta-carotene.

There is some evidence that a diet high in lycopene may reduce the risk of cancer of the prostate as well as other cancers. Lycopene may also help prevent macular degeneration and cataracts.

Sources

Lycopene is not a necessary nutrient. However, like other substances found in fruits and vegetables, it may be very important for optimal health.

Tomatoes are the best source of lycopene. Happily, cooking doesn't destroy lycopene, so pizza sauce is just as good as a fresh tomato. In fact, some studies indicate that cooking tomatoes in oil may provide lycopene in a way that the body can use better,[1,2] although not all studies agree.[3]

Therapeutic Dosages

The optimum dosage for lycopene has not been established. However, one study on lycopene and prostate cancer suggested that about 6.5 mg is an effective daily intake.[4]

Therapeutic Uses

Lycopene may help prevent cancer, particularly cancer of the prostate, but also possibly cancer of the lung, colon, and breast.[5–11] However, the evidence we have for this idea comes from *observational* studies in which researchers analyze people's diets, rather than the more definitive *intervention* trials, in which people are actually given lycopene supplements. In observational trials, it is always possible that other unrecognized factors are at work.

Weak evidence also suggests that lycopene can reduce the risk of cataracts and macular degeneration.[12]

What Is the Scientific Evidence for Lycopene?

Cancer Prevention

Although there are no double-blind studies on lycopene, the results of observational studies are impressive.

One study followed 47,894 men for 4 years.[13] Subjects who ate large amounts of tomatoes or tomato sauce (including that on pizza) had lower rates of prostate cancer. In an evaluation that compared these foods to others that were studied, lycopene appeared to be the common denominator.[14]

Some evidence suggests that lycopene may also help prevent lung, colon, and breast cancer as well.[15] In one study, elderly Americans who ate a diet high in tomatoes had 50%

fewer cancers overall than those who did not.[16] Animal studies have also found some cancer-preventative benefits with lycopene.[17,18]

However, other observational studies have not found lycopene to be the key cancer-fighting ingredient in fruits and vegetables.[19,20] What we really need are large double-blind studies in which people are given either pure lycopene supplements or placebo treatment. Unfortunately, none have yet been performed.

Safety Issues

Although lycopene is a normal part of the diet, there has not been a formal evaluation of lycopene's safety when it is taken as a concentrated supplement. Maximum safe dosages for young children, pregnant or nursing women, or those with severe liver or kidney disease have not been established.

LYSINE

Supplement Forms/Alternate Names
L-Lysine, Lysine Hydrochloride
Principal Proposed Uses
Herpes Simplex (Cold Sores, Genital Herpes)

Lysine is an essential amino acid, one that you need to get from food. Evidence suggests that supplemental lysine may be able to help prevent herpes infections (cold sores and genital herpes), especially when combined with certain dietary changes.

Requirements/Sources

Most people need about 1 g of lysine per day. The requirement may be greater for athletes and people recovering from major injuries, especially burns. The richest sources of lysine are animal proteins such as meat and poultry, but it is also found in dairy products, eggs, and beans.

Therapeutic Dosages

A typical therapeutic dosage of lysine for herpes is 1 g 3 times daily. You can take this as a regular part of your diet in hopes of preventing herpes flare-ups, or, perhaps, at the first sign of an attack. For best results, you should probably restrict your intake of foods that contain a lot of arginine (see Therapeutic Uses).

Therapeutic Uses

Some small studies suggest that regular use of lysine supplements can reduce the number of herpes flare-ups, although other studies have not found the same benefit.[1–6] Lysine has also been proposed as a treatment to take at the onset of a herpes attack, but at least one study has found it to be ineffective for this purpose.[7]

Both cold sores and genital herpes are caused by a virus called *herpes simplex*. After you are first infected, this virus hides in certain nerve cells, and reemerges under times of stress. Test-tube research suggests that lysine fights this virus by blocking arginine, an amino acid the virus needs in order to replicate.[8]

For this reason, lysine may be most effective when used in conjunction with a low-arginine diet. Foods that you should avoid include chocolate, peanuts and other nuts, seeds, and, to a lesser extent, wheat. (See the chapter on arginine for more information about this amino acid.)

What Is the Scientific Evidence for Lysine?

Herpes Simplex

Although the evidence is preliminary and somewhat contradictory, on balance it appears that regular use of lysine supplements might be able to reduce the number and intensity of herpes flare-ups.[9] However, a study evaluating lysine taken only at the onset of a herpes attack found no benefit.[10]

One double-blind placebo-controlled study enrolled 52 participants with a history of herpes flare-ups.[11] While receiving 3 g of L-lysine every day for 6 months, the treatment group experienced an average of 2.4 fewer herpes flare-ups than the placebo group—a significant difference. The lysine group's flare-ups were also significantly less severe and healed faster.

Another double-blind placebo-controlled study on 41 subjects also found improvements in the frequency of attacks.[12] Interestingly, this study found that 1,250 mg of lysine daily worked, but 624 mg did not.

However, other studies, including one that enrolled 79 individuals, found no benefit.[13,14]

Although some are promising, none of these studies are large enough to give conclusive answers. At this point, more evidence is needed to determine whether lysine is an effective treatment for herpes simplex.

Safety Issues

Although lysine is an essential part of the diet, the safety of concentrated lysine supplements has not been well studied. In animal studies, high dosages have caused gallstones and elevated cholesterol levels,[15,16] so you may want to use caution when using lysine if you have either of these problems. Maximum safe dosages for young children, pregnant or nursing women, or those with severe liver or kidney disease have not been established.

MAGNESIUM

Supplement Forms/Alternate Names
Magnesium Chloride, Magnesium Citrate, Magnesium Fumarate, Magnesium Gluconate, Magnesium Malate, Magnesium Oxide, Magnesium Sulfate

Principal Proposed Uses
Migraine Headaches, Noise-Related Hearing Loss, Kidney Stones, Hypertension (High Blood Pressure)

Other Proposed Uses
Atherosclerosis, PMS, Painful Menstruation (Dysmenorrhea), Diabetes, Osteoporosis, Low Blood Sugar, Glaucoma, Fibromyalgia, Fatigue, Low HDL ("Good") Cholesterol, Stroke, Autism

Various Forms of Heart Disease: Mitral Valve Prolapse, Congestive Heart Failure

Asthma

Magnesium is an essential nutrient mineral, meaning that your body needs it for healthy functioning. It is found in significant quantities throughout the body and used for numerous purposes, including muscle relaxation, blood clotting, and the manufacture of ATP (adenosine triphosphate, the body's main energy molecule).

It has been called "nature's calcium channel–blocker." The idea refers to magnesium's ability to block calcium from entering muscle and heart cells. A group of prescription heart medications work in a similar way, although much more powerfully. This may be the basis for magnesium's effects on migraine headaches and high blood pressure.

Magnesium is one of the few essential nutrients for which deficiencies are fairly common. For this reason, it is probably reasonable for most people to take magnesium on general principle, regardless of particular therapeutic use.

Requirements/Sources

Requirements for magnesium increase as we grow and age. The U.S. Recommended Dietary Allowance is as follows

- Infants under 6 months, 30 mg
    6 to 12 months, 75 mg
- Children 1 to 3 years, 80 mg
    4 to 8 years, 130 mg
- Males 9 to 13 years, 240 mg
    14 to 18 years, 410 mg
    19 to 30 years, 400 mg
    31 years and older, 420 mg
- Females 9 to 13 years, 240 mg
    14 to 18 years, 360 mg
    19 to 30 years, 310 mg
    31 years and older, 320 mg
- Pregnant women 18 years and younger, 400 mg
    19 to 30 years, 350 mg
    31 to 50 years, 360 mg
- Nursing women 18 years and younger, 360 mg
    19 to 30 years, 310 mg
    31 to 50 years, 320 mg

In the United States, the average dietary intake of magnesium is significantly lower than it should be.[1,2] Alcohol, surgery, diabetes, certain types of diuretics ("water pills"), estrogen and oral contraceptives, and zinc have been reported to reduce your body's level of magnesium or increase magnesium requirements.[3,4,5] If you are taking potassium or manganese, you may need extra magnesium as well.[6]

While it is sometimes said that calcium interferes with magnesium absorption, it apparently has no significant effect on overall magnesium status.[7,8]

Estrogen (as in estrogen-replacement therapy and oral contraceptives) may decrease blood levels of magnesium by causing the mineral to move into body tissues and bone. For this reason, individuals who don't get enough dietary magnesium may need to take a magnesium supplement.

Kelp is very high in magnesium, as are wheat bran, wheat germ, almonds, and cashews. Other good sources include blackstrap molasses, brewer's yeast (not to be confused with nutritional yeast), buckwheat, and nuts and whole grains. You can also get appreciable amounts of magnesium from collard greens, dandelion greens, avocado, sweet corn, Cheddar cheese, sunflower seeds, shrimp, dried fruit (figs, apricots, and prunes), and many other common fruits and vegetables.

Therapeutic Dosages

A typical supplemental dosage of magnesium ranges from the nutritional needs previously described to as high as 600 mg daily. For premenstrual syndrome (PMS) and dysmenorrhea (painful menstruation), an alternative approach is to start taking 500 to 1,000 mg daily, beginning on day 15 of the menstrual cycle and continuing until menstruation begins.

Magnesium may interfere with the absorption of various other minerals. For this reason it's suggested that those taking magnesium should also take a multimineral supplement.

Therapeutic Uses

Several preliminary studies suggest that regular use of magnesium can help prevent migraine headaches.[9,10,11]

Magnesium may also be useful for protecting the ears against hearing loss caused by exposure to loud noises,[12] reducing the incidence of kidney stones,[13] and perhaps reducing hypertension.[14,15,16] There is also some evidence that magnesium may decrease the atherosclerosis risk caused by hydrogenated oils, margarine-like fats found in many "junk" foods.[17]

Preliminary double-blind trials suggest that magnesium may be useful for dysmenorrhea (menstrual cramps)[18,19] and symptoms of PMS (premenstrual syndrome), including menstrual migraines.[20,21]

Although there is no direct evidence that magnesium helps people with diabetes, such individuals are known to be deficient in magnesium,[22,23,24] and magnesium supplementation may be a good idea on general principle. (However, individuals with severe kidney disease should take magnesium supplements only on their physician's advice.)

Magnesium has also been suggested as a treatment for osteoporosis, low blood sugar, glaucoma, fibromyalgia, fatigue, stroke, low HDL ("good") cholesterol, autism, Alzheimer's disease, angina, attention deficit disorder, periodontal disease, rheumatoid arthritis, and various forms of heart disease including mitral valve prolapse and congestive heart failure. However, there is little to no real evidence that it is effective for these purposes.

Alternative medicine literature frequently mentions magnesium as a treatment for asthma. However, this idea seems to be based entirely on the outdated practice of using intravenous magnesium as an emergency treatment for asthma. When you take something by mouth, it's a very different matter from having it injected into your veins. There is no real evidence that oral magnesium helps asthma, and even some evidence that it does not help.[25]

Warning: Do not self-inject magnesium! See your doctor for such treatment.

Finally, magnesium supplements have been suggested for reducing complications of pregnancy such as preeclampsia, but a double-blind study of 400 pregnant women found no benefit.[26]

What Is the Scientific Evidence for Magnesium?

Migraine Headaches
A recent double-blind study found that regular use of magnesium helps prevent migraine headaches. In this 12-week trial, 81 people with recurrent migraines were given either 600 mg of magnesium daily or placebo.[27] By the last 3 weeks of the study, the treated group's migraines had been reduced by 41.6%, compared to a reduction of 15.8% in the placebo group. The only side effects observed were diarrhea (in about one-fifth of the participants) and, less often, digestive irritation.

Similar results have been seen in other, smaller double-blind studies.[28,29] One study found no benefit,[30] but it has been criticized on many significant points, including using an excessively strict definition of what constituted benefit.[31]

Noise-Related Hearing Loss

One double-blind placebo-controlled study on 300 military recruits suggests that 167 mg of magnesium daily can prevent hearing loss due to exposure to high-volume noise.[32]

Kidney Stones

Magnesium inhibits the growth of calcium oxalate stones in the test tube[33] and decreases stone formation in rats.[34] However, human studies have had mixed results. In one 2-year open study, 56 people taking magnesium hydroxide had fewer recurrences of kidney stones than 34 people not given magnesium.[35] In contrast, a double-blind (and, hence, more reliable) study of 124 individuals found that magnesium hydroxide was essentially no more effective than placebo.[36]

Hypertension (High Blood Pressure)

Magnesium works with calcium and potassium to regulate blood pressure. Several studies suggest that magnesium supplements can reduce blood pressure in people with hypertension,[37–40] although some have not.

Dysmenorrhea

A 6-month, double-blind, placebo-controlled study of 50 women with menstrual pain found that treatment with magnesium significantly improved symptoms.[41] The researchers reported evidence of reduced levels of prostaglandin F_2 alpha, a hormone-like substance involved in pain and inflammation.

Similarly positive results were seen in a double-blind placebo-controlled study of 21 women.[42]

PMS Symptoms

A double-blind placebo-controlled study of 32 women found that magnesium taken from day 15 of the menstrual cycle to the onset of menstrual flow could significantly improve premenstrual mood changes.[43]

Another small double-blind study (20 participants) found that magnesium supplementation can help prevent menstrual migraines.[44]

Safety Issues

In general, magnesium appears to be quite safe when taken at recommended dosages. The most common complaint is loose stools. However, people with severe kidney or heart disease should not take magnesium (or any other supplement) except on the advice of a physician. Maximum safe dosages have not been established for young children or women who are pregnant or nursing. There has been one case of death caused by excessive use of magnesium supplements in a developmentally and physically disabled child.

Magnesium can interfere with the absorption of antibiotics in the tetracycline family.[45] Also, when combined with oral diabetes drugs in the sulfonylurea family (Tolinase, Micronase, Orinase, Glucotrol, Diabinese, DiaBeta), magnesium may cause blood sugar levels to fall more than expected.[46]

⚠ Interactions You Should Know About

If you are taking

- **Potassium supplements**, **manganese**, **diuretics**, **oral contraceptives**, **estrogen-replacement therapy:** You may need extra magnesium.
- **ACE inhibitors**, antibiotics in the **tetracycline** or **quinolone** (e.g., Cipro) families, **Dilantin (phenytoin)**, **H₂ blockers** (e.g., Zantac or Pepcid), **Macrodantin**, or **zinc:** You should take magnesium at a different time of day to avoid absorption problems.
- **Digoxin:** You may need extra magnesium, but magnesium can impair the absorption of digoxin. The solution: take them at least 2 hours apart.
- **Oral diabetes medications** in the sulfonylurea family: Work closely with your physician when taking magnesium to avoid hypoglycemia.

MANGANESE

Supplement Forms/Alternate Names
Manganese Chloride, Manganese Gluconate, Manganese Picolinate, Manganese Sulfate

Principal Proposed Uses
Osteoporosis, Dysmenorrhea (Menstrual Pain)

Other Proposed Uses
Muscle Sprains/Strains, Rheumatoid Arthritis, Epilepsy, Diabetes

---

Our bodies contain only a very small amount of manganese, but this metal is important as a constituent of many key enzymes. The chemical structure of these enzymes is interesting: large protein molecules cluster around a tiny atom of metal.

Manganese plays a particularly important role as part of the natural antioxidant enzyme superoxide dismutase (SOD), which helps fight damaging free radicals. It also helps energy metabolism, thyroid function, blood sugar control, and normal skeletal growth.

Requirements/Sources

Manganese is thought to be an essential nutrient, but the precise daily requirement isn't known. The following daily amounts are considered safe and adequate

- Infants under 6 months, 0.3 to 0.6 mg
    6 to 12 months, 0.6 to 1 mg
- Children 1 to 3 years, 1 to 1.5 mg
    4 to 6 years, 1.5 to 2.0 mg
    7 to 10 years, 2.0 to 3.0 mg
- Adults (and children 11 years and older), 2 to 5 mg

Antacids as well as calcium, iron, copper, magnesium, and zinc supplements can reduce the body's absorption of manganese.[1,2] The best sources of dietary manganese are whole grains, legumes, avocados, grape juice, chocolate, seaweed, egg yolks, nuts, seeds, boysenberries, blueberries, pineapples, spinach, collard greens, peas, and green vegetables.

Therapeutic Dosages

A typical dosage used in studies on manganese is 3 to 6 mg daily. It is sometimes recommended at a much higher dose of 50 to 200 mg daily for 2 weeks following a muscle sprain or strain, but the safety of this dosage is not known.

Therapeutic Uses

Because manganese plays a role in bone metabolism, it has been suggested as a treatment for osteoporosis, a condition in which bone mass deteriorates with age.[3] However, we have no direct evidence that manganese is helpful, except in combination with other minerals.

Manganese has also been suggested for dysmenorrhea (painful menstruation),[4] muscle strains and sprains, and rheumatoid arthritis, but the evidence that it works is very weak.

People with epilepsy have lower-than-normal levels of manganese in their blood.[5] This suggests (but doesn't prove) that manganese supplements might be helpful for epilepsy. Unfortunately, the studies that could prove or disprove this idea haven't been performed. A similar situation exists regarding diabetes, where manganese deficiencies have been noted, but no trials that used manganese supplements have been reported.[6]

What Is the Scientific Evidence for Manganese?

Osteoporosis

Although manganese is known to play a role in bone metabolism, there is no direct evidence that manganese supplements can help prevent osteoporosis. However, one double-blind placebo-controlled study suggests that a combination of minerals including manganese may be helpful.[7]

Fifty-nine women took either placebo, calcium (1,000 mg daily), or calcium plus a daily mineral supplement consisting of 5 mg of manganese, 15 mg of zinc, and 2.5 mg of copper. After 2 years, the group receiving calcium plus minerals showed better bone density than the group receiving calcium alone. But this study doesn't tell us whether it was the manganese or the other minerals that made the difference.

Dysmenorrhea (Menstrual Pain)

One very small double-blind study suggested that 5.6 mg of manganese daily might ease menstrual discomfort.[8] In the same study, a lower dosage of 1 mg daily wasn't effective.

Safety Issues

Manganese appears to be safe when taken at the usual recommended dosage of 6 mg or less daily. However, the safety of higher doses is not known. Very high exposure to manganese (due either to environmental pollution or manganese mining) has resulted in a serious psychiatric disorder known as "manganese madness."

⚠ Interactions You Should Know About

If you are taking

- **Iron**, **copper**, **zinc**, **magnesium**, or **calcium:** You may need extra manganese, and vice versa.
- **Antacids:** You may also need extra manganese.

MEDIUM-CHAIN TRIGLYCERIDES

Supplement Forms/Alternate Names
MCTs
Principal Proposed Uses
Difficulty Digesting Fat (Especially in AIDS), Athletic Performance
Other Proposed Uses
Weight Loss, Epilepsy

Medium-chain triglycerides (MCTs) are fats with an unusual chemical structure that allows the body to digest them easily. Most fats are broken down in the intestine and remade into a special form that can be transported in the blood. But MCTs are absorbed intact and taken to the liver, where they are used directly for energy. In this sense, they are processed very similarly to carbohydrates.

MCTs are different enough from other fats that they can be used as fat substitutes by people (especially those with AIDS), who need calories but are unable to absorb or metabolize normal fats.

MCTs are also popular among athletes as a proposed performance enhancer, although there is little evidence as yet that they really work.

Source

There is no dietary requirement for MCTs. Coconut oil, palm oil, and butter contain up to 15% MCTs (plus a lot of other fats). You can also buy MCTs as purified supplements.

Therapeutic Dosages

MCTs can be eaten as salad oil or used in cooking. When taken as an athletic supplement, dosages in the neighborhood of 85 mg daily are common.

Therapeutic Uses

Preliminary evidence suggests that MCTs are a useful fat substitute for those who have trouble digesting fat. This includes people with serious diseases such as AIDS who need to find a way to gain weight.[1,2] It might also be helpful for those who have trouble digesting fatty foods because they lack the proper enzymes (pancreatic insufficiency).[3]

MCTs are also popular among athletes as a concentrated source of easily utilized energy.[4,5,6]

More controversially, MCTs have been used to promote ketosis, a fat-burning state that can cause weight loss,[7] and also improve certain symptoms of epilepsy. In ketosis, the body burns its stored fat for energy. It ordinarily occurs in starvation, but it can be produced on purpose by eating few or no carbohydrates and consuming protein and fat instead. However, intentional ketosis has potential health risks and it is controversial.

What Is the Scientific Evidence for Medium-Chain Triglycerides?

Fat Malabsorption

A double-blind placebo-controlled study on 24 men and women with AIDS suggests that MCTs can help improve AIDS-related fat malabsorption.[8] In this disorder, fat is not digested; it passes unchanged through the intestines, and the body is deprived of calories as well as fat-soluble vitamins.

The study subjects were split into two groups: One received a liquid diet containing normal fats, whereas the other group received mostly MCTs. After 12 days, the participants on the MCT formula showed significantly less fat in their stool and better fat absorption than the other group.

Another double-blind study found similar results in 24 men with AIDS-related fat malabsorption.[9]

The body depends on enzymes from the pancreas to digest fat. In one study, individuals with inadequate pancreatic function due to chronic pancreatitis appeared to be better able to absorb MCTs than ordinary fatty acids.[10] However, this didn't turn out to mean much on a practical basis, because without taking extra digestive enzymes they could only just barely absorb the MCTs; whereas, if they took digestive enzymes, they absorbed ordinary fats as well as MCTs without difficulty.

Athletic Performance

MCTs have been proposed as an "ergogenic aid," an energy-boosting supplement to enhance athletic performance. During intense exercise, your body first burns up available energy from the blood (in the form of glucose) and then starts to use energy stored in the form of a larger carbohydrate called *glycogen*. When the glycogen is depleted, exhaustion begins to set in.

One solution to this is *carbo-loading*, the practice of taking large doses of carbohydrates prior to exercise in order to increase glycogen stores. Athletes can also sip carbohydrate-loaded drinks during exercise.

MCTs may provide an alternative. Like other fats, they provide more energy per ounce than carbohydrates; but unlike normal fats, this energy can be released rapidly.[11]

A very small study compared MCTs and carbohydrates as performance boosters for 6 trained cyclists. The athletes took a 4.3% MCT beverage, a 10% carbohydrate beverage, or a drink containing both 4.3% MCTs and 10% carbohydrate.[12] Researchers found a slight advantage to the combination drink. Another study on 12 cyclists also suggested that MCTs plus carbohydrates enhanced performance.[13] However, a recent small study found no benefit with MCTs, and the researchers felt that there was some impairment of performance due to a sensation of bloating.[14] Larger studies are necessary to discover whether MCTs are really as useful for athletes as some of its proponents claim.

Safety Issues

MCTs are thought to be quite safe, but the safety of using them as a general fat substitute has not been established. Some people who consume MCTs, especially on an empty stomach, experience annoying (but not severe) abdominal cramps and bloating. People with diabetes should not use MCTs (or any other supplement) without a doctor's supervision. The safety of MCTs in young children, pregnant or nursing women, or people with serious kidney or liver disease has not been established.

MELATONIN

Principal Proposed Uses
Sleep Disorders: Insomnia, Jet Lag

Other Proposed Uses
Cancer (As an Addition to Conventional Therapy), Strengthening the Immune System, Preventing Heart Disease, Fighting Aging, Reducing Anxiety Before Surgery, Epilepsy in Children

---

Melatonin is a natural hormone that regulates sleep. During daylight, the pineal gland in the brain produces an important neurotransmitter called *serotonin*. (A neurotransmitter is a chemical that relays messages between nerve cells.) But at night, the pineal gland stops producing serotonin and instead makes melatonin. This melatonin release helps trigger sleep.

The production of melatonin varies according to the amount of light you're exposed to; for example, your body produces more melatonin in a completely dark room than in a dimly lit one.

Melatonin hit the news in 1995. Not only was it recommended as a treatment for insomnia and jet lag, but for various theoretical reasons it was also described as a "wonder hormone" that could fight cancer, boost the immune system, prevent heart disease, and generally make you live longer. But all we really know is that it helps people whose natural sleep cycle has been disturbed, such as travelers suffering from jet lag and swing-shift workers.

Contrary to earlier reports, it does not appear that melatonin levels naturally decline with age.[1]

Sources

Melatonin is not a nutrient. However, travelers and workers on rotating or late shifts can experience sleep disturbances that seem to be caused by changing melatonin levels.

You can boost your melatonin production naturally by getting thicker blinds for the bedroom windows or wearing a night mask. You can also take melatonin tablets.

Therapeutic Dosages

Melatonin is typically taken half an hour before bedtime for the first 4 days after traveling; however, the optimum dose is not clear. According to some studies, 0.5 mg is sufficient, while other studies have found benefits for insomnia only at 10 times the dose (5 mg).[2]

Melatonin is available in two forms: quick-release and slow-release. There is some debate as to which one is better.

Therapeutic Uses

Reasonably good evidence tells us that melatonin can help people with jet lag or other similar sleep disturbances adjust to a new schedule.[3] Melatonin also appears to be helpful for people with other types of insomnia, although the evidence is not strong.[4–9]

Melatonin may also help individuals who have been using conventional sleeping pills and wish to quit.[10]

A recent preliminary study suggests that melatonin may be useful for epilepsy in children.[11]

Highly preliminary evidence suggests that melatonin may be useful for some forms of cancer when combined with conventional anticancer treatment.[12–15] The explanation for this possible effect is unknown, and it may not be true for certain forms of chemotherapy. It is strongly recommended that you consult with your oncologist if you wish to take melatonin during chemotherapy.

Based on fairly theoretical findings, it has been suggested that melatonin can boost the immune system, prevent heart disease, and help you live longer.[16–19]

One double-blind study found that melatonin was useful for reducing anxiety prior to surgery.[20]

What Is the Scientific Evidence for Melatonin?

Sleep Disorders

There is good evidence that melatonin can help you fall asleep when your bedtime rhythm has been disturbed. For example, one double-blind placebo-controlled study enrolled 320 people and followed them for 4 days after plane travel. The participants were divided into four groups and given a daily dose of 5 mg of standard melatonin, 5 mg of slow-release melatonin, 0.5 mg of standard melatonin, or placebo.[21] The group that received 5 mg of standard melatonin slept better, took less time to fall asleep, and felt more energetic and awake during the day than the other three groups.

According to one review of the literature, melatonin treatment for jet lag is most effective for those who have crossed a significant number of time zones, perhaps eight.[22] One study on travelers found no benefit, but it may be that the change in time zones experienced by these travelers wasn't great enough to require melatonin.[23]

Mixed results have been seen in other studies involving swing-shift workers and people with ordinary insomnia.[24–31]

Many people taking conventional sleeping pills (most of which are in the benzodiazepine family) find it difficult to quit. If you try to stop taking your medication, you may experience severe insomnia or interrupted sleep. A double-blind placebo-controlled study of 34 individuals who regularly used such medications found that melatonin at a dose of 2 mg nightly (controlled-release formulation) could help them discontinue the use of the drugs.[32]

Note: There can be risks in discontinuing benzodiazepine drugs. Consult your physician for advice.

Anxiety Prior to Surgery

Relaxing sedative medications are often used prior to surgery to help reduce the anxiety while waiting for surgery to begin. A double-blind placebo-controlled study of 75 women waiting for surgery compared melatonin against the standard drug midazolam.[33] Although midazolam was more effective, melatonin was definitely superior to placebo, and patients appeared to like each one equally. One advantage of melatonin was that it did not cause amnesia.

Cancer

Melatonin has been used with conventional anticancer therapy in more than a dozen clinical studies. Results have been surprisingly good, although this research must be considered preliminary. For example, a double-blind study on 30 people with advanced brain tumors suggested that melatonin might prolong life and also improve the quality of life.[34] Participants received standard radiation treatment with or without 20 mg daily of melatonin. After 1 year, 6 of 14 individuals in the melatonin group were still alive, compared with just 1 of 16 from the control group. The melatonin group also had fewer side effects due to the radiation treatment—a notable improvement in their quality of life.

Improvements in symptoms and a possible reduction of mortality were also seen in other studies.[35,36] Melatonin appears to work by increasing levels of the body's own tumor-fighting proteins, known as *cytokines*.[37]

Safety Issues

Melatonin is probably safe for occasional use, but its safety when used on a regular basis remains unknown. Keep in mind that melatonin is not truly a food supplement but a hormone.

As we know from other hormones used in medicine, such as estrogen and cortisone, harmful effects can take years to appear. Hormones are powerful substances that have many subtle effects in the body, and we're far from understanding them fully.

Because melatonin promotes sleep, you should not drive or operate machinery for several hours after taking it. In addition, melatonin may impair balance.[38] Also, based on theoretical ideas of how melatonin works, some authorities specifically recommend against using it in people with depression, schizophrenia, autoimmune diseases, and other serious illnesses. Maximum safe dosages for young children, pregnant or nursing women, or those with serious liver or kidney disease have not been established.

METHIONINE

Supplement Forms/Alternate Names
L-Methionine

Principal Proposed Uses
There are no well-documented uses for methionine.

Other Proposed Uses
Urinary Tract Infections, "Liver Support"

Methionine is an essential amino acid—one of the building blocks of proteins and peptides that your body cannot manufacture from other chemicals. The body uses methionine to manufacture creatine and uses the sulfur in methionine for normal metabolism and growth.

One preliminary study suggests that methionine can prevent bacteria from sticking to urinary tract cells,[1] which may make it useful for preventing bladder infections. (Cranberry juice is thought to help reduce the incidence of bladder infections in a similar fashion.)

Requirements/Sources

Depending on your body weight, you need between 800 and 1,000 mg of methionine daily for normal health. Deficiency is unlikely, because enough methionine is generally available from the diet.

Meat, fish, dairy products, and other high-protein foods are good sources of methionine.

Therapeutic Dosages

A proper therapeutic dosage of methionine has not been determined. One study relating to urinary tract infections used a dosage of 500 mg 3 times daily.

Therapeutic Uses

Because it seems to discourage bacteria from sticking to the wall of the bladder, methionine has been suggested as a treatment for recurrent bladder infections.[2] However, there is as yet little direct evidence that it works.

One study on rats suggests that methionine might protect the liver against acetaminophen (e.g., Tylenol) poisoning.[3] Based on this, it has been proposed as a generally helpful substance—what our great-grandparents might have called a "tonic"—for the liver. However, in this particular study the action of methionine was more to fight acetaminophen specifically than to protect the liver in general. There is much better evidence that the herb milk thistle is a general liver protectant.

Is the Scientific Evidence for Methionine?

Bladder Infection

The clinical evidence for this use of methionine is based primarily on one study, a preliminary open trial that tested methionine against the standard treatment in 33 women with recurrent urinary tract infections. The dosage used in this study was 500 mg 3 times daily. Researchers found no infections in the methionine group during the 26-month study period.[4] Although methionine did not reduce the number of bacteria in the urinary tract, it appeared to lessen the bacteria's ability to latch on to cells.

Safety Issues

Methionine is thought to be generally safe. However, the maximum safe dosages for young children, pregnant or nursing women, or those with serious liver or kidney disease have not been established.

⚠ Interactions You Should Know About

If you are taking **methionine**, make sure to get enough folate, vitamin B_6, and vitamin B_{12}.[5]

N-ACETYL CYSTEINE (NAC)

Principal Proposed Uses
Angina Pectoris (in Combination with Conventional Treatment)
Other Proposed Uses
Acute Respiratory Distress Syndrome, Bronchitis, Emphysema,
Chemotherapy Aid

N-acetyl cysteine (NAC) is a specially modified form of the dietary amino acid cysteine. NAC may help break up mucus, which is the basis for using it in respiratory conditions. It also helps the body make the important antioxidant enzyme glutathione. However, the only well-documented uses of NAC are for conditions too serious for self-treatment.

Sources

There is no daily requirement for NAC, and it is not found in food.

Therapeutic Dosages

Optimal levels of NAC have not been determined. The amount used in studies has varied from 250 to 1,500 mg daily.

Therapeutic Uses

Mixed evidence suggests that NAC may be helpful for people who take the drug nitroglycerin for angina (the chest pain associated with heart disease).[1-4] However, severe headaches may develop as a side effect. NAC may also be helpful in a life-threatening condition called acute respiratory distress syndrome.[5] Finally, very high dosages of NAC are used in hospitals as a conventional treatment for acetaminophen poisoning.

Note: Do not attempt to self-treat angina, acute respiratory distress syndrome, or acetaminophen poisoning! Medical supervision is absolutely essential because of the very real risk of death in these conditions.

NAC is sometimes recommended as a treatment for bronchitis and emphysema, based on its mucus-thinning effects, and as an aid for enduring chemotherapy. However, there is no solid scientific evidence that it is effective for these conditions.

What Is the Scientific Evidence for N-Acetyl Cysteine (NAC)?

Angina Pectoris

Angina pectoris is a squeezing feeling in the chest caused by inadequate blood supply to the heart. It can be a precursor of heart attacks. People with angina often use the drug nitroglycerin to relieve symptoms. One 4-month, double-blind, placebo-controlled study of 200 individuals with heart disease found that the combination of nitroglycerin and NAC significantly reduced the incidence of heart attacks and other severe heart problems.[6] NAC alone and nitroglycerin alone were not as effective. The only problem was that the combination of nitroglycerin and NAC caused severe headaches in many participants. This effect has been seen in other studies as well.[7]

NAC may also help in cases of nitroglycerin tolerance, a condition in which the drug becomes less effective over time. In a small double-blind study of 32 people with angina, tolerance developed in 15 of 16 individuals who took nitroglycerin only, but in just 5 of 16 individuals who took nitroglycerin plus 2 g of NAC daily.[8] However, other studies have found no benefit.[9]

Acute Respiratory Distress Syndrome

A double-blind placebo-controlled clinical trial compared the effectiveness of NAC, Procysteine (a synthetic cysteine building-block drug), and placebo in 46 people with a condition called *acute respiratory distress syndrome*.[10] This catastrophic lung condition can be caused when an unconscious person inhales his or her own vomit. Both NAC and Procysteine reduced the severity of the condition in some people (as compared with placebo). However, overall it did not reduce the number of deaths.

Safety Issues

NAC appears to be a very safe supplement when taken alone, although one study in rats suggests that 60 to 100 times the normal dose can cause liver injury.[11]

As mentioned earlier, the combination of nitroglycerin and NAC causes severe headaches. Safety in young children, women who are pregnant or nursing, and individuals with severe liver or kidney disease has not been established.

⚠ Interactions You Should Know About

If you are taking **nitroglycerin**, NAC may cause severe headaches.

NADH

Supplement Forms/Alternate Names
Nicotinamide Adenine Dinucleotide
Principal Proposed Uses
There are no well-documented uses for NADH.
Other Proposed Uses
Alzheimer's Disease, Chronic Fatigue Syndrome, Depression, Parkinson's Disease, Exercise Performance Enhancement

NADH, short for *nicotinamide adenine dinucleotide*, is an important cofactor, or "assistant," that helps enzymes in the work they do throughout the body. NADH particularly plays a role in the production of energy. It also participates in the production of L-dopa, which the body turns into the important neurotransmitter dopamine.

Based on these basic biochemical facts, NADH has been suggested as a treatment for Alzheimer's disease, Parkinson's disease, chronic fatigue syndrome, and depression and as a sports supplement. However, there isn't enough scientific evidence to prove or disprove its usefulness for any of these conditions.

Sources

Healthy bodies make all the NADH they need, using vitamin B_3 (also known as niacin, or nicotinamide) as a starting point. The highest concentration of NADH in animals is found in muscle tissues, which means that meat might be a good source—were it not that most of the NADH in meat is destroyed during processing, cooking, and digestion. In reality, we don't get much NADH from our food.

Therapeutic Dosages

The typical dosage for supplemental NADH ranges from 5 to 50 mg daily.

Therapeutic Uses

Supplemental NADH has been proposed as a treatment for Alzheimer's disease, chronic fatigue syndrome, depression, and Parkinson's disease. It has also been tried as an athletic performance enhancer. However, although a few studies have been performed on these uses,[1–4] none were designed in such a way as to produce scientifically meaningful results.

Safety Issues

NADH appears to be quite safe when taken at a dosage of 5 mg daily or less. However, formal safety studies have not been completed, and safety in young children, pregnant or nursing women, or those with severe liver or kidney disease has not been established.

OPCs (OLIGOMERIC PROANTHOCYANIDINS)

Supplement Forms/Alternate Names
Grape Seed Extract, Pine Bark Extract, Procyanidolic Oligomers (PCOs)

Principal Proposed Uses
Strengthening Blood Vessels/ Reducing Inflammation: Varicose Veins, Hemorrhoids, Edema (Swelling) Following Injury or Surgery, Easy Bruising

Other Proposed Uses
Aging Skin, Cancer Prevention, Diabetic Neuropathy, Diabetic Retinopathy, Atherosclerosis Prevention, Macular Degeneration, Allergies, Poor Night Vision, Liver Cirrhosis

One of the bestselling herbal products of the early 1990s was an extract of the bark of French maritime pine. This substance consists of a family of chemicals known scientifically as oligomeric proanthocyanidin complexes (OPCs) or procyanidolic oligomers (PCOs). Similar substances are also found in grape seed.

The modern use of OPCs is closely linked to an event in 1534, when a French explorer and his crew were trapped by ice in the Saint Lawrence River. Many of the men were saved from scurvy by a Native American who suggested they make tea from the needles and bark of a local pine tree. Over 400 years later, Jacques Masquelier of the University of Bordeaux came across this story and decided to investigate the constituents of pine trees. In 1951, he extracted OPCs from the bark of the maritime pine, and found that they could duplicate many of the functions of vitamin C. Later, he found an even better source of OPCs in grape seed, which is their major source in France today.

Like the anthocyanosides found in bilberry (to which they are closely related), OPCs appear to stabilize the walls of blood vessels, reduce inflammation, and generally support tissues containing collagen and elastin.[1–4] OPCs are also strong antioxidants. Vitamin E defends against fat-soluble oxidants and vitamin C neutralizes water-soluble ones, but OPCs are active against both types.[5,6,7]

Evidence suggests that OPCs can reduce the discomfort and swelling of varicose veins and decrease the edema (swelling) that often follows injury or surgery. On the basis of much weaker evidence, OPCs are also popular for preventing heart disease, revitalizing aging skin, and reducing the tendency toward easy bruising.

Sources

Like other flavonoids, OPCs aren't necessary for life, although they may prove to be important for optimal health.

OPCs aren't a single chemical, but a group of closely related compounds. Several food sources contain similar chemicals: red wine, cranberries, blueberries, bilberries, tea (green and black), black currant, onions, legumes, parsley, and the herb hawthorn. However, most OPC supplements are made from either grape seed or the bark of the maritime pine. Grape seed is the preferred source in France, where this supplement was originally popularized, and is a more economical source than pine bark.

Therapeutic Dosages

For use as a general antioxidant—much as you might use vitamin E or vitamin C (see the chapters on vitamins E and C)—50 mg of OPCs daily are sufficient. A higher dosage of 150 to 300 mg daily is generally used for treating specific diseases such as varicose veins. Grape seed OPCs are just as good and much less expensive than the maritime pine source.

Therapeutic Uses

The best-documented use of OPCs is to treat venous insufficiency, a condition closely related to varicose veins. It refers to the situation when blood pools in the legs, causing aching, pain, heaviness, swelling, fatigue, and unsightly visible veins. Fairly good preliminary evidence suggests that OPCs can relieve the pain and swelling of venous insufficiency.[8,9,10] OPCs probably cannot make visible varicose veins disappear, but regular use might help prevent new ones from developing. Other approaches to varicose veins include horse chestnut, gotu kola, and bromelain. On the basis of their evidence for varicose veins, OPCs are often recommended as a treatment for hemorrhoids as well.

There is also some evidence that OPCs can be useful for the swelling that often follows injuries or surgery.[11,12,13] OPCs appear to speed the disappearance of swelling, presumably by strengthening damaged blood and lymph vessels that are leaking fluid.

For similar reasons, OPCs may also be helpful for people who bruise easily due to fragile blood vessels. **Note:** Keep in mind that there may be medical causes for easy bruising that require more specific treatment.

OPCs in cream form are a popular treatment for aging skin, on the theory that by repairing elastin and collagen they will return skin to a more youthful appearance. However, there is no solid evidence as yet that they are effective for this purpose.

On the basis of preliminary evidence, regular use of OPCs has been proposed as a measure to prevent cancer, diabetic neuropathy and diabetic retinopathy (side effects of diabetes), heart disease, macular degeneration (the major cause of age-related blindness), as well as a treatment for allergies (hay fever), impaired night vision, and liver cirrhosis. However, much more research needs to be performed to discover whether these potential benefits are real.

What Is the Scientific Evidence for OPCs (Oligomeric Proanthocyanidins)?

Considerable evidence tells us that OPCs protect and strengthen collagen and elastin—proteins found in cartilage, tendons, blood vessels, and muscle.[14-19] There is also no question that OPCs are strong antioxidants, more powerful than either vitamin E or vitamin C by some measures.[20] The medicinal effects of OPCs are believed to be due to some combination of these properties.

Venous Insufficiency (Varicose Veins)

There is fairly good preliminary evidence for the use of OPCs to treat people with symptoms of venous insufficiency.

A double-blind placebo-controlled study of 92 subjects found that OPCs, taken at a dose of 100 mg 3 times daily, significantly improved major symptoms, including heaviness, swelling, and leg discomfort.[21] Over a period of 1 month, 75% of the participants treated with OPCs improved substantially. This result doesn't seem quite so impressive when you note that significant improvement was also seen in 41% of the placebo group; nonetheless, OPCs still did significantly better than placebo.

A placebo-controlled study that enrolled 364 individuals with varicose veins found that treatment with OPCs produced results superior to those of placebo.[22] Unfortunately, the rather incomplete report available on this study does not describe the statistical analysis of the results, nor whether physicians were blinded.

Finally, a double-blind study of 50 people with varicose veins of the legs found that doses of 150 mg per day of OPCs were more effective in reducing symptoms and signs than another natural treatment: the bioflavonoid diosmin, widely used in Europe for this condition.[23]

Edema After Surgery or Injury

Breast cancer surgery often leads to swelling of the arm. A double-blind placebo-controlled study of 63 post-operative breast cancer patients found that 600 mg of OPCs daily for 6 months reduced edema, pain, and peculiar sensations known as paresthesias.[24] Also, in a double-blind placebo-controlled study of 32 "face-lift" patients who were followed for 10 days, edema disappeared much faster in the treated group.[25]

Another 10-day, double-blind, placebo-controlled study enrolling 50 participants found that OPCs improved the rate at which edema disappeared following sports injuries.[26]

Night Vision

One interesting, 6-week, controlled (but not blinded) study evaluated the ability of grape seed OPCs to improve night vision in normal subjects.[27,28] In this trial of 100 healthy volunteers, those who received 200 mg per day of OPCs showed improvements in night vision and glare recovery as compared to untreated subjects.

Atherosclerosis

Although there are no reliable human studies, animal evidence suggests that OPCs can slow or reverse atherosclerosis.[29-32] This suggests (but definitely does not prove) that OPCs might be helpful for preventing heart disease.

Safety Issues

OPCs have been extensively tested for safety and are generally considered to be essentially nontoxic.[33] Side effects are rare, but when they do occur they are limited to occasional allergic reactions and mild digestive distress. However, maximum safe dosages for young children, pregnant or nursing women, or those with severe liver or kidney disease have not been established.

OPCs may have some anticoagulant properties when taken in high doses, and should be used only under medical supervision by individuals on blood-thinner drugs, such as Coumadin (warfarin) and heparin.

⚠ Interactions You Should Know About

If you are taking **Coumadin (warfarin)**, **heparin**, **Trental (pentoxifylline)**, or **aspirin**, high doses of OPCs might cause a risk of excessive bleeding.

ORNITHINE ALPHA-KETOGLUTARATE

Principal Proposed Uses
There are no documented uses for ornithine alpha-ketoglutarate.
Other Proposed Uses
Athletic Performance Enhancer

Ornithine alpha-ketoglutarate (OKG) is manufactured from two amino acids, ornithine and glutamine. OKG is not found in food, although its two building blocks are.

Animal studies suggest that OKG may prevent the breakdown of muscle, which has led to the suggestion that it may be helpful for athletes in training.

Sources

The amino acids that make up OKG are found in high-protein foods such as meat, fish, and dairy, but OKG itself is not found in foods. Supplements are available in tablet or pill form.

Therapeutic Dosages

Athletes have taken up to 35 g daily of OKG.

Therapeutic Uses

OKG is widely used by athletes in the hope that it will increase their muscle development in training. However, there is practically no foundation for this belief, other than two rather theoretical studies in rats.[1,2]

Safety Issues

OKG appears to be safe. However, as with all supplements used in multigram doses, it is important to purchase a reputable product, because a contaminant present even in small percentages could add up to a real problem. The maximum safe dosages for young children, women who are pregnant or nursing, or those with serious liver or kidney disease have not been established.

PABA (PARA-AMINOBENZOIC ACID)

Principal Proposed Uses
There are no well-documented uses for PABA.

Other Proposed Uses
Scleroderma, Peyronie's Disease, Male Infertility, Vitiligo

Para-aminobenzoic acid (PABA) is best known as the active ingredient in sunblock. This use of PABA is not really medicinal: like a pair of sunglasses, PABA physically blocks ultraviolet rays when it is applied to the skin.

There are, however, some proposed medicinal uses of oral PABA supplements. PABA is sometimes suggested as a treatment for various diseases of the skin and connective tissue, as well as for male infertility. However, most of the clinical data on PABA comes from very old studies, some from the early 1940s.

Sources

PABA is not believed to be an essential nutrient. Nonetheless, it is found in foods, mainly in grains and meat. Small amounts of PABA are usually present in B vitamin supplements as well as in some multiple vitamins.

Therapeutic Dosages

A typical therapeutic dosage of PABA is 300 to 400 mg daily. Some studies have used much higher dosages. However, serious side effects have been found in dosages above 8 g daily (see Safety Issues). You probably shouldn't take more than 400 mg daily except on medical advice.

Therapeutic Uses

PABA has been suggested as a treatment for scleroderma, a disease that creates fibrous tissue in the skin and internal organs.[1,2] However, a small double-blind study found it ineffective.[3]

PABA has also been suggested for other diseases in which abnormal fibrous tissue is involved, such as Peyronie's disease, a condition in which the penis becomes bent owing to the accumulation of such tissue.[4,5,6] However, no double-blind studies have yet been performed.

Based on one small World War II–era study, PABA has been suggested for treating male infertility as well as vitiligo, a condition in which patches of skin lose their pigment, resulting in pale blotches. However, this study didn't have a control group, so its results aren't meaningful.[7] Ironically, a recent study suggests that high dosages of PABA can cause vitiligo (see Safety Issues).

Safety Issues

PABA is probably safe when taken at a dosage up to 400 mg daily. Possible side effects at this dosage are minor, including skin rash and loss of appetite.[8]

Higher doses are a different story, however. There has been one reported case of severe liver toxicity in a woman taking 12 g daily of PABA.[9] Fortunately, her liver recovered completely after she discontinued her use of this supplement. Also, a recent study suggests that 8 g daily of PABA can cause vitiligo, the patchy skin disease described previously.[10]

Clearly, there are questions that need to be answered about the safety of high-dose PABA therapy. You shouldn't take more than 400 mg daily except under medical supervision.

PABA can interfere with certain medications, including sulfa antibiotics.[11]

Safety in young children, pregnant or nursing women, or those with serious liver or kidney disease has not been determined.

⚠ Interactions You Should Know About

If you are taking **sulfa antibiotics** such as **Bactrim** or **Septra**, do not take PABA supplements except on medical advice.

PANTOTHENIC ACID AND PANTETHINE

Principal Proposed Uses
High Triglycerides/High Cholesterol

Other Proposed Uses
Rheumatoid Arthritis, Athletic Performance, Stress

Note: Pantothenic acid is often sold as calcium pantothenate. Pantethine, a special form of pantothenic acid, appears to have some unique properties. Regular pantothenic acid cannot be used as a substitute for pantethine.

The body uses pantothenic acid (better known as vitamin B_5) to make proteins as well as other important chemicals needed to metabolize fats and carbohydrates. Pantothenic acid is also used in the manufacture of hormones, red blood cells, and *acetylcholine*, an important neurotransmitter (signal carrier between nerve cells). As a supplement, pantothenic acid has been proposed as a treatment for rheumatoid arthritis, an athletic performance enhancer, and an "antistress" nutrient.

In the body, pantothenic acid is converted to a related chemical known as pantethine. For reasons that are not clear, pantethine supplements (but not pantothenic acid supplements) appear to reduce levels of both triglycerides and cholesterol in the blood.

Requirements/Sources

The word *pantothenic* comes from the Greek word meaning "everywhere," and pantothenic acid is indeed found in a wide range of foods. For this reason, pantothenic acid deficiency is rare. Although an exact daily requirement is not known, the

Estimated Safe and Adequate Daily Dietary Intake is as follows

- Infants under 6 months, 2 mg
     6 to 12 months, 3 mg
- Children 1 to 3 years, 3 mg
     4 to 6 years, 3 to 4 mg
     7 to 10 years, 4 to 5 mg
- Males and females 11 years and older, 4 to 7 mg

Brewer's yeast, torula (nutritional) yeast, and calf liver are excellent sources of pantothenic acid. Peanuts, mushrooms, soybeans, split peas, pecans, oatmeal, buckwheat, sunflower seeds, lentils, rye flour, cashews, and other whole grains and nuts are good sources as well, as are red chili peppers and avocados. Pantethine is not found in foods in appreciable amounts.

Therapeutic Dosages

For lowering cholesterol and triglycerides, the typical recommended dosage of pantethine is 300 mg 3 times daily. Dosages of pantothenic acid as high as 660 mg 3 times daily are sometimes recommended for people with arthritis.

Therapeutic Uses

Quite a few small studies suggest that pantethine may lower blood levels of triglycerides and, to a lesser extent, cholesterol.[1,2,3] In general, elevated cholesterol is more harmful than elevated triglycerides. However, some people have only modestly elevated cholesterol but very high triglycerides, so pantethine may be especially useful for them. It also may be particularly helpful for people with diabetes who need to lower their triglyceride and/or cholesterol levels.[4–7]

Pantothenic acid has been proposed as a treatment for rheumatoid arthritis, but the evidence for this use is quite weak.[8,9]

Pantothenic acid is also recommended as an athletic performance enhancer, but there is no good evidence at all that it works. It is also sometimes referred to as an antistress nutrient because it plays a role in the function of the adrenal glands, but whether it really helps the body withstand stress is not known.

What Is the Scientific Evidence for Pantothenic Acid and Pantethine?

High Triglycerides/High Cholesterol

Several small studies suggest (but do not prove) that pantethine can reduce total blood triglycerides and perhaps cholesterol as well.[10,11,12] For example, a double-blind placebo-controlled study followed 29 people with high cholesterol and triglycerides for 8 weeks.[13] The dosage used was 300 mg 3 times daily, for a total daily dose of 900 mg. In this study, subjects taking pantethine experienced a 30% reduction in blood triglycerides, a 13.5% reduction in LDL ("bad") cholesterol, and a 10% rise in HDL ("good") cholesterol. However, for reasons that are unclear, some studies have found no benefit.[14,15]

Several other studies have specifically studied the use of pantethine to improve cholesterol and triglyceride levels in people with diabetes and found it effective.[16–19]

These findings are supported by experiments in rabbits, which show that pantethine may prevent the buildup of plaque in major arteries.[20] We don't know how pantethine works in the body.

Rheumatoid Arthritis

There is weak evidence for using pantothenic acid to treat rheumatoid arthritis. One observational study found 66 people with rheumatoid arthritis had less pantothenic acid in their blood than 29 healthy people. The more severe the arthritis, the lower the blood levels of pantothenic acid were.[21] However, this result doesn't prove that pantothenic acid supplements can effectively reduce any of the symptoms of rheumatoid arthritis.

To follow up on this finding, researchers then conducted a small placebo-controlled trial involving 18 subjects to see whether pantothenic acid would help. This study found that 2 g daily of pantothenic acid (in the form of calcium pantothenate) reduced morning stiffness, pain, and disability significantly better than placebo.[22] However, a study this small doesn't mean much on its own. More research is needed.

Safety Issues

No significant side effects have been reported for pantothenic acid or pantethine, used by themselves or with other medications. However, maximum safe dosages for young children, pregnant or nursing women, or people with serious liver or kidney disease have not been established.

PHENYLALANINE

Supplement Forms/Alternate Names
D-Phenylalanine, DL-Phenylalanine, L-Phenylalanine
Principal Proposed Uses
Depression
Other Proposed Uses
Chronic Pain: Rheumatoid Arthritis, Muscle Pain, Osteoarthritis
Vitiligo, Attention Deficit Disorder

Phenylalanine occurs in two chemical forms: *L-phenylalanine,* a natural amino acid found in proteins; and its mirror image, *D-phenylalanine,* a form synthesized in a laboratory. Some research has involved the L-form, others the D-form, and still others a combination of the two known as DL-phenylalanine.

In the body, phenylalanine is converted into another amino acid called tyrosine. Tyrosine in turn is converted into L-dopa, norepinephrine, and epinephrine, three key neurotransmitters (chemicals that transmit signals between nerve cells). Because some antidepressants work by raising levels of norepinephrine, various forms of phenylalanine have been tried as a possible treatment for depression.

D-phenylalanine (but not L-phenylalanine) has been proposed to treat chronic pain. It blocks *enkephalinase,* an enzyme that may act to increase pain levels in the body. Phenylalanine (various forms) has also been suggested as a treatment for vitiligo, a disease characterized by abnormal white blotches of skin due to loss of pigmentation.

Requirements/Sources

L-phenylalanine is an essential amino acid, meaning that we need it for life and our bodies can't manufacture it from other chemicals. It is found in protein-rich foods such as meat, fish, poultry, eggs, dairy products, and beans. Provided you eat enough protein, you are likely to get enough L-phenylalanine for your nutritional needs. There is no nutritional need for D-phenylalanine.

Therapeutic Dosages

When used as a treatment for depression, L-phenylalanine is typically started at a dosage of 500 mg daily, and then gradually increased to 3 to 4 g daily.[1] However, side effects may develop at dosages above 1,500 mg daily (see Safety Issues).

D- or DL-phenylalanine may be used for depression as well, but the typical dosage is much lower: 100 to 400 mg daily.[2]

For the treatment of chronic pain, usual recommended dosages of D-phenylalanine are as high as 2,500 mg daily.

It is best not to take your phenylalanine supplement at the same time as a high-protein meal, as it may not be absorbed well.

Therapeutic Uses

Preliminary studies suggest that both the L- and D-forms of phenylalanine may be helpful for depression.[3,4]

Weak evidence suggests that D-phenylalanine may be useful for chronic pain,[5] such as rheumatoid arthritis, muscle pain, and osteoarthritis, but this conclusion has been contested.[6,7,8]

A preliminary double-blind study found that the combination of phenylalanine and ultraviolet radiation might be helpful for vitiligo.[9]

Although it is sometimes proposed as a treatment for attention deficit disorder, phenylalanine taken alone does not appear to be helpful for attention deficit disorder.[10,11] Some proponents claim that it works better when combined with tyrosine, glutamine, and gamma-aminobutyric acid (GABA), but this has not been proven.

What Is the Scientific Evidence for Phenylalanine?

Depression

A pair of double-blind studies have found that D- or DL-phenylalanine is as effective as imipramine, a standard antidepressant drug, and that it may take effect much more quickly. The larger of the two studies compared the effectiveness of D-phenylalanine at 100 mg daily against the same daily dose of imipramine.[12] Sixty people with depression were randomly assigned to take either imipramine or D-phenylalanine for 30 days. The results in both groups were statistically equivalent, meaning that phenylalanine was about as effective as imipramine. D-phenylalanine worked more rapidly, however, producing significant improvement in only 15 days. Like most antidepressant drugs, imipramine requires several weeks to take effect.

The other double-blind study followed 27 individuals, half of whom received DL-phenylalanine (150 to 200 mg daily) and the other half imipramine (100 to 150 mg daily).[13] When they were reevaluated after 30 days, both groups had improved by a statistically equal amount. Very preliminary studies have also found benefits with L-phenylalanine.[14,15]

Unfortunately, there have been no good studies comparing any form of phenylalanine against placebo. This is too bad, since without such evidence we can't be sure that the supplement is actually effective.

Chronic Pain

The use of D-phenylalanine to treat pain is primarily based on a study involving 43 individuals with chronic pain, mostly due to arthritis.[16] However, this was not a double-blind study, and it suffered from other flaws as well.[17]

A small double-blind study reportedly found evidence for the effectiveness of D-phenylalanine in chronic pain,[18] but a careful look at the math involved undermined that conclusion.[19] Another small study found no benefits.[20]

Safety Issues

Although most people do not report side effects from any type of phenylalanine, daily doses near or above 1,500 mg of L-phenylalanine can reportedly cause anxiety, headache, and even mildly elevated blood pressure.[21]

The long-term safety of phenylalanine in any of its forms is not known. Both L- and D-phenylalanine must be avoided by those with the rare metabolic disease phenylketonuria (PKU).

The safety of high dosages of L-phenylalanine, or any dosage of D-phenylalanine, has not been established for young children, pregnant or nursing women, or those with severe liver or kidney disease.

There are some indications that the combined use of phenylalanine with antipsychotic drugs might increase the risk of developing the long-term side effect known as tardive dyskinesia.[22,23]

⚠ Interactions You Should Know About

If you are taking **antipsychotic medications**, do not use phenylalanine.

PHOSPHATIDYLSERINE

Principal Proposed Uses
Alzheimer's Disease, Age-Related Memory Loss
Other Proposed Uses
General Improvement of Mental Performance, Depression, Enhancement of Athletic Training

---

Phosphatidylserine (fos-fah-TIDE-ul-ser-een), or PS for short, is a member of a class of chemical compounds known as *phospholipids*. PS is an essential component in all our cells; specifically, it is a major component of the cell membrane. The cell membrane is a kind of "skin" that surrounds living cells. Besides keeping cells intact, this membrane performs vital functions such as moving nutrients into cells and pumping waste products out of them. PS plays an important role in many of these functions.

Good evidence suggests that PS can help declining mental function and depression in the elderly, and it is widely used for this purpose in Italy, Scandinavia, and other parts of Europe. PS has also been marketed as a "brain booster" for people of all ages, said to sharpen memory and increase thinking ability.

Recently, PS has been marketed as a sports supplement, said to help bodybuilders and power athletes develop larger and stronger muscles.

Sources

Your body makes all the PS it needs. However, the only way to get a therapeutic dosage of PS is to take a supplement.

PS was originally manufactured from the brains of cows, and all the studies described here used this form. However, because animal brain cells can harbor viruses, that form is no longer available, and most PS today is made from soybeans.

According to some experts, soy-based PS is just as effective as PS made from cows' brains.[1–5] However, not everyone agrees.[6]

Phosphatidylserine can also be manufactured from cabbage, but in one study the results with this form of the supplement were not impressive.[7]

Therapeutic Dosages

For the purpose of improving mental function, PS is usually taken in dosages of 100 mg 2 to 3 times daily. After maximum effect is achieved, the dosage can sometimes be reduced to 100 mg daily without losing benefit. PS can be taken with or without meals.

When taking PS for sports purposes, athletes may use as much as 800 mg daily.

Therapeutic Uses

Impressive evidence from numerous double-blind studies suggests that PS is an effective treatment for Alzheimer's disease and other forms of age-related mental decline.[8–17]

PS is widely marketed as a treatment for ordinary age-related memory loss, and there is some evidence that it might work. Keep in mind that in studies of severe mental decline, PS was equally effective whether the cause was Alzheimer's disease or something entirely unrelated (multiple small strokes). This certainly suggests that PS may have a positive impact on the brain that is not specific to any one condition. From this observation, it is not a great leap to suspect that it might make it useful for much less severe problems with memory and mental function, such as those that seem to occur in nearly all of us who are older than 40. Indeed, one double-blind study did find that phosphatidylserine could improve mental function in individuals with relatively mild age-related memory loss.[18]

PS may also be helpful for depression.[19,20,21]

Recently, PS has become popular among athletes who hope it can help them build muscle more efficiently. This use is based on modest evidence that PS slows the release of cortisol following heavy exercise.[22,23,24] Cortisol is a hormone that causes muscle tissue to break down. For reasons that are unclear, the body produces increased levels of cortisol after heavy exercise. Strength athletes believe that this natural cortisol release works against their efforts to rapidly build muscle mass and hope that PS will help them advance more quickly. However, this idea has not been proven.

What Is the Scientific Evidence for Phosphatidylserine?

Alzheimer's Disease and Other Forms of Dementia

Overall, the evidence for PS in dementia is quite strong. Double-blind studies involving a total of over 1,000 people suggest that phosphatidylserine (at least the type from cow's brain) is an effective treatment for Alzheimer's disease and other forms of dementia.

The largest of these studies followed 494 elderly subjects in northeastern Italy over a course of 6 months.[25] All suffered from moderate to severe mental decline, as measured by standard tests. Treatment consisted of either 300 mg daily of PS or placebo. The group that took PS did significantly better in both behavior and mental function than the placebo group. Symptoms of depression also improved.

These results agree with those of numerous smaller double-blind studies involving a total of over 500 people with Alzheimer's and other types of age-related dementia.[26–33]

Ordinary Age-Related Memory Loss

There is some evidence that PS can also help people with ordinary age-related memory loss. In one double-blind study that enrolled 149 individuals with memory loss but not dementia, phosphatidylserine provided significant benefits as compared with placebo.[34] Individuals with the most severe memory loss showed the most improvement.

Athletic Performance

Weak evidence suggests that PS might decrease the release of the hormone cortisol after intense exercise.[35] Among its many effects, cortisol acts to break down muscle tissue—

exactly the opposite of the effect desired by a strength athlete or bodybuilder. This double-blind placebo-controlled study on 11 intensely trained athletes found that 800 mg of PS taken daily reduced the cortisol rise by 20% as compared with placebo.[36] Another small study on 9 nonathletic males found that daily doses of 400 and 800 mg of PS reduced cortisol levels after exercise by 16% and 30%, respectively.[37] Another study found that phosphatidylserine could relieve some overtraining symptoms, including muscle soreness, possibly due to effects on cortisol.[38,39,40]

However, there is as yet no direct evidence to support the claims that PS actually helps athletes build muscles more quickly and with less training effort.

Safety Issues

Phosphatidylserine is generally regarded as safe when used at recommended dosages. Side effects are rare, and when they do occur they usually consist of nothing much worse than mild gastrointestinal distress.[41] However, the maximum safe dosages for young children, pregnant or nursing women, or those with severe liver or kidney disease have not been established.

PS is sometimes taken with ginkgo because they both appear to enhance mental function. However, some caution might be in order: Ginkgo is a "blood thinner," and PS might be one as well. Together, the two supplements might interfere with normal blood clotting enough to cause problems. Although this is still hypothetical, we do have reason to believe that PS can enhance the effect of heparin, a very strong prescription blood thinner.[42]

Keep in mind, too, that Alzheimer's disease and other types of severe age-related mental impairment are too serious to treat on your own with PS or any other supplement. In some cases, the symptoms of these diseases may be a sign of other serious conditions. If you suspect that you or a loved one may have a severe age-related mental impairment, see your doctor for diagnosis and treatment.

⚠ Interactions You Should Know About

If you are taking

- **Prescription blood thinners**, such as **heparin** or **Coumadin (warfarin)**: Do not use phosphatidylserine except on a physician's advice.
- **Ginkgo**: Taking phosphatidylserine at the same time might conceivably "thin" the blood too much.

POTASSIUM

Supplement Forms/Alternate Names
Chelated Potassium (Potassium Aspartate, Potassium Citrate), Potassium Bicarbonate, Potassium Chloride
Principal Proposed Uses
Hypertension (High Blood Pressure)

Potassium is a mineral found in many foods and supplements. But you will never see pure potassium in a health food store or pharmacy—it's a highly reactive metal that bursts into flame when exposed to water! The potassium you eat, or take as a supplement, is composed of potassium atoms bound to other nonmetallic substances—less exciting, perhaps, but chemically stable.

Potassium is one of the major *electrolytes* in your body, along with sodium and chloride. Potassium and sodium work together like a molecular seesaw: when the level of one goes up, the other goes down. All together, these three dissolved minerals play an intimate chemical role in every function of your body.

The most common use of potassium supplements is to make up for potassium depletion caused by diuretic drugs. These medications are often used to help regulate blood pressure, but by depleting the body of potassium they may inadvertently make blood pressure harder to control.

Requirements/Sources

Potassium is an essential mineral that we get from many common foods. The minimum requirement of potassium for children ranges from 1,000 to 2,300 mg daily; adults should receive 1,600 to 2,000 mg daily.

True potassium deficiencies are rare except in cases of prolonged vomiting or diarrhea, or with the use of diuretic drugs.

However, in one sense potassium deficiency is common, at least when compared to the amount of sodium we receive in our diets. It is probably healthy to take in at least five times as much potassium as sodium (and perhaps 50 to 100 times as much). But the standard American diet contains twice as much sodium as potassium. Therefore, taking extra potassium may be a good idea in order to balance the sodium we consume to such excess.

Bananas, orange juice, potatoes, avocados, lima beans, cantaloupes, peaches, tomatoes, flounder, salmon, and cod all contain more than 300 mg of potassium per serving. Other good sources include chicken, meat, and various other fruits, vegetables, and fish.

Over-the-counter potassium supplements typically contain 99 mg of potassium per tablet. There is some evidence that, of the different forms of potassium supplements, potassium citrate may be most helpful for those with high blood pressure.[1]

Research indicates that it is important to get enough magnesium, too, when you are taking potassium.[2] It might be wise to take extra vitamin B_{12} as well.[3]

Therapeutic Dosages

When used by physicians, potassium is usually measured according to meqs (milliequivalents) rather than the more common mg (milligrams). A typical therapeutic dosage of potassium is between 10 and 20 meq (about 200 to 400 mg), taken 3 to 4 times daily.

Therapeutic Uses

Potassium appears to be helpful for hypertension, especially among individuals who eat too much salt.[4,5]

What Is the Scientific Evidence for Potassium?

High Blood Pressure

According to a review of 33 double-blind studies, potassium supplements can produce a slight but definite drop in blood pressure.[6] However, two large studies found no benefit.[7,8] The explanation is probably that potassium is only slightly helpful. When a treatment has only a small effect, it's not unusual for some studies to show no effect while others find a modest benefit. It's possible that potassium may only help people who are at least a bit deficient in this mineral.

Evidence suggests that potassium supplements may be most effective for people who eat too much salt.[9]

Safety Issues

As an essential nutrient, potassium is safe when taken at appropriate dosages. If you take a bit too much, your body will simply excrete it in the urine. However, people who have severe kidney disease or are taking a type of medication called a "potassium-sparing diuretic" cannot excrete potassium normally, and should consult a physician before taking a potassium supplement. (For other drug interactions, see Interactions You Should Know About.)

Potassium pills can cause injury to the esophagus if they get stuck on the way down, so make sure to take them with plenty of water.

⚠ Interactions You Should Know About

If you are taking

- **Loop diuretics** or **thiazide diuretics:** You may need more potassium.
- **ACE inhibitors** (e.g., captopril, lisinopril, enalapril), **potassium-sparing diuretics** (e.g., triamterene or spironolactone): You should not take potassium except on the advice of a physician.

- **Tetracycline antibiotics:** You should take potassium supplements at a different time of day to avoid absorption problems.
- **Potassium:** You may need extra magnesium and vitamin B_{12}.

PREGNENOLONE

Principal Proposed Uses
There are no well-documented uses for pregnenolone.

Other Proposed Uses
Memory Enhancement, Age-Related Hormone Decline, Alzheimer's Disease, Menopausal Symptoms, Adrenal Disease, Parkinson's Disease, Osteoporosis, Fatigue, Stress, Depression, Rheumatoid Arthritis, Nerve Injury, Weight Loss

Pregnenolone has been called "the grandmother of all steroid hormones." The body manufactures it from cholesterol, and then uses it to make testosterone, cortisone, progesterone, estrogen, DHEA, androstenedione, aldosterone, and all other hormones in the "steroid" family.

One reason given for using pregnenolone is that the level of many of these hormones declines with age. By taking pregnenolone supplements, proponents say, you can keep all your hormones at youthful levels. However, pregnenolone levels themselves don't decline with age,[1] and there is no indication that taking extra pregnenolone will increase the levels of any other hormones. Furthermore, even if it did, that doesn't mean using pregnenolone is a great idea.

Steroid hormones are powerful substances, and they can cause harm as well as benefit. Long-term use of cortisone causes severe osteoporosis; estrogen can increase the risk of cancer; and anabolic steroids (used by athletes) may cause liver problems and stress the heart. We really have very little idea what long-term consequences the use of pregnenolone might entail.

Actually, it is ironic that pregnenolone is legally classified as a "dietary supplement" at all. Pregnenolone is not a nutrient. It is a drug, just as estrogen, cortisone, and aldosterone are drugs. We recommend not using it until we know more about what it really does.

Sources

Pregnenolone is not normally obtained from foods. Your body manufactures it from cholesterol. Supplemental pregnenolone is made synthetically in a chemical laboratory from substances found in soybeans.

Therapeutic Dosages

A typical recommended dosage of pregnenolone is 30 mg daily, but some studies have used as much as 700 mg.

Therapeutic Uses

If you browse the Internet or read health magazines, you'll find pregnenolone described as a treatment for an enormous list of health problems, including memory loss, Alzheimer's disease, menopausal symptoms, adrenal disease, Parkinson's disease, osteoporosis, fatigue, stress, depression, rheumatoid arthritis, and nerve injury. It is also supposed to help you lose weight, improve your brain power, and make you feel young again. However, like so many overhyped new supplements, there is very little scientific evidence for any of these uses.

Studies involving rats suggest that pregnenolone may enhance memory,[2,3] but there have been no human studies.

Safety Issues

Pregnenolone is a powerful hormone, not a nutrient we would naturally get in our food. You should approach this supplement with caution, as if it were a drug—for all intents and purposes, it is a drug. It would be best to consult your doctor before taking it. Pregnenolone is definitely not recommended for children, pregnant or nursing women, or those with liver or kidney disease.

PROTEOLYTIC ENZYMES

Supplement Forms/Alternate Names
Bromelain, Chymotrypsin, Digestive Enzymes, Pancreatin, Papain, Trypsin

Principal Proposed Uses
Digestive Aid, Sports Injuries

Other Proposed Uses
Shingles (Herpes Zoster), Food Allergies, Rheumatoid Arthritis, Other Autoimmune Diseases

Proteolytic enzymes help you digest the proteins in food. Although your body produces these enzymes in the pancreas, certain foods also contain proteolytic enzymes.

Papaya and pineapple are two of the richest plant sources, as attested by their traditional use as natural "tenderizers" for meat. Papain and bromelain are the respective names for the proteolytic enzymes found in these fruits. The enzymes made in your body are called trypsin and chymotrypsin.

The primary use of proteolytic enzymes is as a digestive aid for people who have trouble digesting proteins. However, for reasons that are not clear, they also seem to help bruises and other traumas heal faster, which has made them popular in Europe as a treatment for sports injuries. They may also help reduce the pain of shingles.

Many practitioners of alternative medicine believe that proteolytic enzymes can be helpful for a wide variety of other health conditions, including food allergies and autoimmune diseases. However, there is little to no scientific evidence as yet that they really work for these problems.

Sources

You don't need to get proteolytic enzymes from food, because the body manufactures them (primarily trypsin and chymotrypsin). However, deficiencies in proteolytic enzymes do occur, usually resulting from diseases of the pancreas.

Symptoms include abdominal discomfort, gas, indigestion, poor absorption of nutrients, and passing undigested food in the stool.

For use as a supplement, trypsin and chymotrypsin are extracted from the pancreas of various animals. You can also purchase bromelain extracted from pineapple stems and papain made from papayas.

Therapeutic Dosages

When you purchase an enzyme, the amount is expressed not only in grams or milligrams but also in *activity units* or *international units*. These terms refer to the enzyme's potency (i.e., its digestive power). There is more than one way to measure this.

Bromelain dosages are measured in MCUs (milk-clotting units) or GDUs (gelatin-dissolving units). High-potency bromelain preparations contain at least 2,000 MCUs (or 1,333 GDUs) per gram. Some health authorities recommend taking 3,000 MCUs of bromelain 3 times daily.

Dosages of pancreatic extract are rated by an "X" factor: 5X pancreatin is five times stronger than a certain standard pancreatin preparation. If you use pancreatic enzyme extract, a dosage of 0.5 to 1.5 g of 9X pancreatin with each meal is probably sufficient. If you take a lower-strength formulation, you will need a higher dosage.

Proteolytic enzymes can be broken down by stomach acid. To prevent this from happening, supplemental enzymes are often coated with a substance that doesn't dissolve until it reaches the intestine. Such a preparation is called "enteric coated."

Therapeutic Uses

The most obvious use of proteolytic enzymes is to assist digestion.

In addition, some evidence suggests that these enzymes might be able to improve the rate of healing of sports injuries.[1,2] (For another approach, see OPCs [Oligomeric

Proanthocyanidins].) We don't really know how they work, but it probably isn't by affecting digestion. The explanation may lie in evidence that proteolytic enzymes can be absorbed whole[3] and may produce a variety of effects in the body.

One study suggests that proteolytic enzymes might be helpful for the treatment of the painful condition known as shingles (herpes zoster).[4]

Proteolytic enzymes may also help reduce symptoms of food allergies, presumably by digesting the food so well that there is less to be allergic to.

Proteolytic enzymes have also been proposed as a treatment for rheumatoid arthritis and other autoimmune diseases. According to a theory popular in alternative medicine circles, these diseases may be made worse by whole proteins from foods leaking into the blood and causing an immune reaction. Digestive enzymes may help foil this so-called "leaky gut" problem. (For another approach, see Glutamine.) However, there is no real evidence as yet to substantiate this use.

What Is the Scientific Evidence for Proteolytic Enzymes?

Sports Injuries

Two small double-blind studies, involving a total of about 50 athletes, found that treatment with proteolytic enzymes significantly speeded healing of bruises and other mild athletic injuries, as compared to placebo.[5,6]

Safety Issues

Proteolytic enzymes are believed to be quite safe, although there are some concerns that they might further damage the exposed tissue in an ulcer (by partly digesting it). One proteolytic enzyme, pancreatin, may interfere with folate absorption (see Folate).[7]

⚠ Interactions You Should Know About

If you take the proteolytic enzyme **pancreatin**, you may need extra folate.

PYRUVATE

Supplement Forms/Alternate Names
Calcium Pyruvate, Dihydroxyacetone Pyruvate (DHAP), Magnesium Pyruvate, Potassium Pyruvate, Sodium Pyruvate

Principal Proposed Uses
Weight Reduction

Other Proposed Uses
Enhancing Athletic Endurance

Pyruvate supplies the body with pyruvic acid, a natural compound that plays important roles in the manufacture and use of energy. Pyruvate supplements have become popular with bodybuilders and other athletes, based on claims that pyruvate can reduce body fat and enhance the ability to use energy efficiently. However, at the present time, there is only preliminary evidence that it really works.

Sources

Pyruvate is not an essential nutrient, since your body makes all it needs. But it can be found in food, with an average diet supplying anywhere from 100 mg to 2 g daily. Apples are the best source: a single apple contains about 450 mg of pyruvate. Beer and red wine contain about 75 mg per serving.

Therapeutic dosages are usually much higher than what you can get from food: You'd have to eat almost 70 apples a day to get the proper amount! To use pyruvate for therapeutic purposes, you must take a supplement.

Although most products on the market contain only (or almost only) pyruvate, some also contain small amounts of a related compound, dihydroxyacetone, which the body converts to pyruvate. The combination of the two products is known as DHAP.

Therapeutic Dosages

A typical therapeutic dosage of pyruvate is 30 g daily.

Therapeutic Uses

Evidence from several small double-blind studies suggests that pyruvate may enhance weight loss.[1-4] Preliminary evidence also suggests that pyruvate may slightly increase an athlete's capacity for endurance exercise.[5,6] Unfortunately, these studies were all too small for the results to mean very much.

What Is the Scientific Evidence for Pyruvate?

Weight Reduction

In one double-blind placebo-controlled study, 34 people trying to lose weight were given either placebo or a dosage of pyruvate ranging from 22 to 44 g daily.[7] The treatment group lost significantly more weight.

Smaller studies have found similar benefits.[8,9,10]

Safety Issues

Both pyruvate and dihydroxyacetone appear to be quite safe, aside from mild side effects such as occasional stomach upset and diarrhea. However, maximum safe dosages for children, women who are pregnant or nursing, or those with liver or kidney disease have not been established.

Keep in mind that, because such enormous doses of pyruvate are used, if a contaminant were present even in very small percentages there could be harmful results. For this reason, you should make sure to use a high-quality product.

QUERCETIN

Supplement Forms/Alternate Names
Quercetin Chalcone

Principal Proposed Uses
There are no well-documented uses for quercetin.

Other Proposed Uses
Asthma, Allergies (Hay Fever), Eczema, Hives, Heart Disease Prevention, Stroke Prevention, Cancer Prevention

You may have heard of the "French paradox." The French diet is very high in fat and cholesterol (just think of *pate de fois gras* and croissants), yet France has one of the world's lowest rates of heart disease. One theory for this discrepancy is that another major player in the French diet—red wine—protects the arteries of the heart.

A natural antioxidant found in red wine, quercetin protects cells in the body from damage by free radicals (naturally occurring but harmful substances). Heart disease and high cholesterol are thought to be at least partly caused by free radical damage to blood vessels, so it makes sense that quercetin might help protect against heart attacks and strokes. Quercetin belongs to a class of water-soluble plant coloring agents called *bioflavonoids*, a type of nutrient that we're learning more about all the time. Although they don't seem to be essential to life, it's likely that we need them for optimal health.

Another intriguing finding is that quercetin may help prevent immune cells from releasing *histamine*, the chemical that initiates the itching, sneezing, and swelling of an allergic reaction. Based on this very preliminary research, quercetin is often recommended as a treatment for allergies and asthma.

Sources

Quercetin is not an essential nutrient. It is found in red wine, grapefruit, onions, apples, black tea, and, in lesser amounts, in leafy green vegetables and beans. However, to get a therapeutic dosage, you'll have to take a supplement.

Quercetin supplements are available in pill and tablet form. One problem with them, however, is that they don't seem to be well absorbed by the body. A special form called quercetin chalcone appears to be better absorbed.

Therapeutic Dosages

A typical dosage is 200 to 400 mg 3 times daily. Quercetin may be better absorbed if taken on an empty stomach.

Therapeutic Uses

The most popular use of quercetin is as a treatment for allergic conditions such as asthma, hay fever, eczema, and hives. This use is based on test-tube research showing that quercetin prevents certain immune cells from releasing histamine, the chemical that triggers an allergic reaction.[1] It also may block other substances involved with allergies.[2] But we have no evidence as yet that taking quercetin supplements will reduce your allergy symptoms.

Very preliminary evidence also suggests that quercetin might help prevent heart disease and strokes.[3-7]

Test-tube and animal research also suggests that quercetin might have anticancer properties.[8-12]

An animal study found that quercetin might protect rodents with diabetes from forming cataracts.[13] Another intriguing finding of test-tube research is that quercetin seems to prevent a wide range of viruses from infecting cells and reproducing once they are inside cells. One study found that quercetin produced this effect against herpes simplex, polio virus, flu virus, and respiratory viruses.[14,15] However, none of this research tells us whether humans taking quercetin supplements can hope for the same benefits. Much more research needs to be done on the use of quercetin for these conditions.

Safety Issues

Quercetin appears to be quite safe. However, at one point concerns were raised that it might cause cancer. Quercetin "fails" a standard laboratory test called the Ames test, which is designed to identify chemicals that might be carcinogenic. However, a bad showing on the Ames test does not definitely mean a chemical causes cancer. Other evidence suggests that quercetin does not cause cancer, and may in fact help prevent cancer.[16,17,18] Maximum safe dosages for young children, women who are pregnant or nursing, or those with serious liver or kidney disease have not been established.

RED YEAST RICE

Supplement Forms/Alternate Names
Hong Qu, Monascus purpureus
Principal Proposed Uses
High Cholesterol

Red yeast rice is a traditional Chinese substance that is made by fermenting a type of yeast called *Monascus purpureus* over rice. This product (called Hong Qu) has been used in China since at least 800 A.D. as a food and also as a medicinal substance. Recently, it has been discovered that this ancient Chinese preparation contains at least 11 naturally occurring substances similar to prescription drugs in the "statin" family, such as Mevacor and Pravachol. These medications are highly effective at reducing cholesterol.

What Is Red Yeast Rice Used for Today?

Presumably because it contains substances similar or identical to statin drugs, red yeast rice appears to be effective at lowering cholesterol. However, because of potential risks, it should be used only under physician supervision.

What Is the Scientific Evidence for Red Yeast Rice?

A recent major U.S. study on red yeast rice was conducted at the UCLA School of Medicine.[1] This was a 12-week double-blind placebo-controlled trial involving 83 healthy participants (46 men and 37 women, aged 34 to 78 years) with high cholesterol levels. One group was given the recommended dose of red yeast rice, while the other group received a placebo. Both groups were instructed to consume a low-fat diet similar to the American Heart Association Step 1 diet.

The results showed that red yeast rice was significantly more effective than placebo. In the treated group, average total cholesterol (mg/dL) fell by about 18% by 8 weeks. During the same time period, LDL ("bad") cholesterol decreased by 22% and triglycerides by 11%. There was little to no

improvement in the placebo group. HDL ("good") cholesterol did not change in either group during the study.

Similar or even better results have been seen in other U.S.
and Chinese studies using various forms of red yeast rice.[2,3]

Dosage

Because red yeast rice products can vary widely in their
strength, please refer to the labeling for appropriate dosage.

Safety Issues

While there have been no serious adverse reactions reported
in the studies of red yeast rice, some minor side effects have
been reported. In the large study of 446 people, heartburn
(1.8%), bloating (0.9%), and dizziness (0.3%) were all mentioned. Formal toxicity studies in rats and mice, giving doses
up to 125 times the normal human dose for 3 months,
showed no toxic effects, according to unpublished information on file with one of the manufacturers of red yeast rice.[4]

However, because red yeast rice contains ingredients
similar to the statin drugs, there is a theoretical risk of the
same side effects and risks that are seen with those drugs.
These include elevated liver enzymes, damage to skeletal
muscle, and increased risk of cancer.

Red yeast rice should not be combined with erythromycin, other statin drugs, the class of drugs called "fi-
brates," or high-dose niacin (for lowering cholesterol).
Serious side effects have occurred when statin drugs were
combined with these medications.

Grapefruit juice can cause a significant and possibly dangerous increase in blood levels of statin drugs. For this reason, grapefruit juice should be avoided when taking red yeast
rice.

This product should not be used by pregnant or nursing
mothers, or those with severe liver or kidney disease except
on a physician's advice.

⚠ Interactions You Should Know About

If you are taking

- **Erythromycin**, cholesterol-lowering drugs in the **statin** or fibrate family, or high-dose **niacin**: Do not take red yeast rice.
- **Red yeast rice**: Do not drink grapefruit juice.

RESVERATROL

Supplement Forms/Alternate Names
Grape Skin

Principal Proposed Uses
There are no well-documented uses for resveratrol.

Other Proposed Uses
Heart Disease, Cancer Prevention

You may have heard of the "French paradox." The national diet of France includes a lot of butter, cream, meat, and other high-fat, high-cholesterol foods suspected to be bad for the heart. Yet France has one of the world's *lowest* rates of heart disease. The leading theory attempting to explain this puzzle suggests that the French are somehow protected from cardiovascular disease because they drink red wine.

Resveratrol is an ingredient of red wine that may be at least partly responsible for this beneficial effect. (Quercetin is another such ingredient. See Quercetin.) Resveratrol is a *polyphenol,* a natural antioxidant that protects cells against dangerous, naturally occurring substances known as free radicals.

Test-tube and observational studies have linked resveratrol to reduced rates of heart disease and cancer. Unfortunately, there hasn't been any clinical research on human beings yet, but the attention resveratrol has been getting via news stories on the "French Paradox" might lead to clinical studies in the near future.

Sources

Resveratrol is not an essential nutrient. It is found in red wine as well as in red grape skins and seeds and purple grape juice. Peanuts also contain a small amount of resveratrol. Resveratrol supplements are available as well.

Therapeutic Dosages

Because there haven't been any clinical studies, the optimal therapeutic dosage hasn't been established for resveratrol. Based on animal studies, a reasonable therapeutic dosage of resveratrol might be about 500 mg daily.

Therapeutic Uses

Very preliminary evidence suggests that resveratrol may help prevent heart disease,[1–4] although some studies have not been favorable.[5,6,7]

Test-tube studies also suggest that resveratrol might have a number of properties that might make it helpful for preventing cancer.[8–13]

Safety Issues

Resveratrol appears to be quite safe according to the research done thus far, but full safety studies have not been performed. Maximum safe dosages for children, pregnant or nursing women, or those with severe liver or kidney disease have not been determined.

SAMe (S-ADENOSYLMETHIONINE)

Supplement Forms/Alternate Names
Ademetionine, S-Adenosylmethionine, SAM

Principal Proposed Uses
Osteoarthritis, Depression

Other Proposed Uses
Liver Disease, Parkinson's Disease, Fibromyalgia

S-adenosylmethionine is quite a mouthful; the abbreviation *SAMe* (pronounced "Sammy") is easier to say. Its chemical structure and name are derived from two materials you may have heard about already: methionine, a sulfur-containing amino acid; and adenosine triphosphate (ATP), the body's main energy molecule.

SAMe was discovered in Italy in 1952. It was first investigated as a treatment for depression, but along the way it was accidentally noted to improve arthritis symptoms—a kind of positive "side effect." SAMe is presently classed with glucosamine and chondroitin as a potential "chondroprotective" agent, one that can go beyond treating symptoms to actually slowing the progression of arthritis. However, this exciting possibility has not yet been proven.

Unfortunately, SAMe is an extraordinarily expensive supplement at present. Full dosages can easily cost more than $200 per month.

Sources

The body makes all the SAMe it needs, so there is no dietary requirement. However, deficiencies in methionine, folate, or vitamin B_{12} can reduce SAMe levels. SAMe is not found in appreciable quantities in foods, so it must be taken as a supplement. It's been suggested that the supplement TMG (see TMG) might indirectly increase SAMe levels and provide similar benefits, but this effect has not been proven.

Therapeutic Dosages

A typical full dosage of SAMe is 400 mg taken 3 to 4 times per day. If this dosage works for you, take it for a few weeks and then try reducing the dosage. As little as 200 mg twice daily may suffice to keep you feeling better once the full dosage has "broken through" the symptoms.

However, some people develop mild stomach distress if they start full dosages of SAMe at once. To get around this, you may need to start low and work up to the full dosage gradually.

Recently, SAMe has come on the U.S. market at a recommended dosage of 200 mg twice daily. This dosage labeling makes SAMe appear more affordable (if you're only taking 400 mg per day, you'll spend only about a third of what you'd pay for the proper dosage), but it is unlikely that SAMe will actually work when taken at such a low dosage.

Therapeutic Uses

A substantial amount of evidence suggests that SAMe can be an effective treatment for osteoarthritis, the "wear and tear" type of arthritis that many people develop as they get older.[1] However, the supplements glucosamine and chondroitin are much less expensive and just as well documented. (For more information on natural options for arthritis, see Glucosamine and Chondroitin.)

Several small studies suggest that SAMe can be helpful for depression.[2]

This supplement may also be helpful for certain liver conditions such as liver cirrhosis, pregnancy-related jaundice, and Gilbert's syndrome.[3-10] Additionally, SAMe may help the painful muscle condition known as fibromyalgia.[11,12]

SAMe might be helpful for individuals with Parkinson's disease. It has been found to reduce the depression so commonly associated with the disease.[13] In addition, the drug levodopa, used for Parkinson's disease, depletes the body of SAMe.[14,15] This suggests that taking extra SAMe might be helpful. However, it is also possible that SAMe could interfere with the effect of levodopa, requiring an increase in dosage.

What Is the Scientific Evidence for SAMe (S-Adenosylmethionine)?

Although there have been many studies of SAMe, a substantial percentage of them involved intravenous use of the supplement instead of the oral form. Here we discuss only the evidence for SAMe when it is taken orally.

Osteoarthritis

A substantial body of scientific evidence supports the use of SAMe to treat osteoarthritis.[16] Double-blind studies involving a total of more than a thousand participants suggest that SAMe is about as effective as standard anti-inflammatory drugs.

For example, a double-blind placebo-controlled Italian study tracked 732 people taking SAMe, naproxen (a standard anti-inflammatory drug), or placebo.[17] After 4 weeks, participants taking SAMe or naproxen showed about the same level of benefit as compared with those in the placebo group.

Another double-blind study compared SAMe with the anti-inflammatory drug piroxicam.[18] A total of 45 individuals were followed for 84 days. The two treatments proved equally effective. However, the SAMe-treated individuals maintained their improvement long after the treatment was stopped, whereas those on piroxicam quickly started to hurt again. Similarly long-lasting results have been seen with glucosamine and chondroitin. This pattern of response suggests that these treatments are somehow making a deeper impact on osteoarthritis than simply relieving symptoms. However, while we have direct evidence that glucosamine and chondroitin can slow the progression of osteoarthritis, we do not know for sure that SAMe offers the same benefit.

In other double-blind studies, oral SAMe has also shown equivalent benefits to various doses of indomethacin, ibuprofen, and naproxen.[19,20,21]

Depression

SAMe's antidepressant activity was first reported in 1976.[22] Since then, several small double-blind studies involving a total of more than 200 individuals have found oral SAMe to be an effective treatment for depression.[23-29] Some of these studies compared SAMe with placebo, while others used a control group given another antidepressant drug. Unfortunately, none of these trials enrolled more than 60 participants, and many of the studies suffered from significant design flaws. Solid evidence that SAMe is effective for depression will require a large (100 participants or more), double-blind, placebo-controlled trial.

Liver Disease

A 2-year double-blind study of 123 individuals with liver disease found that treatment with SAMe improved survival time in those with less advanced disease.[30] Other studies showed benefits in a variety of other liver conditions, including liver toxicity caused by oral contraceptives, pregnancy-related jaundice, and Gilbert's syndrome.[31–37]

Parkinson's Disease

Evidence suggests that levodopa (the drug used to treat Parkinson's disease) can reduce brain levels of SAMe.[38,39] This depletion may contribute to the side effects of levodopa treatment, as well as the depression sometimes seen with Parkinson's disease. One study found that SAMe taken orally improved depression without changing the effectiveness of levodopa.[40] However, it is also possible that over time taking extra SAMe could interfere with levodopa's effectiveness.

Safety Issues

SAMe appears to be quite safe, according to both human and animal studies.[41–44] The most common side effect is mild digestive distress. However, SAMe does not actually damage the stomach.[45]

Like other substances with antidepressant activity, SAMe might trigger a manic episode in those with bipolar disease (manic-depressive illness).[46,47,48]

Safety in young children, pregnant or nursing women, or those with severe liver or kidney disease has not been established.

There may be risks involved in combining SAMe with standard antidepressants.[49] Consult your doctor before combining SAMe with any antidepressant medication.

⚠ Interactions You Should Know About

If you are taking

- Standard antidepressants, including **MAO inhibitors**, **SSRIs**, and **tricyclics:** Do not take SAMe except on a physician's advice.
- **Medications for manic-depressive disease:** Do not take SAMe except on a physician's advice.
- **Drugs that are "excreted by conjugation":** It is possible that use of SAMe may require you to increase your medication dose.[50] Ask your pharmacist for advice.
- **Levodopa** for Parkinson's disease: SAMe might help relieve the side effects of this drug. However, it might also reduce its effectiveness over time.

SELENIUM

Supplement Forms/Alternate Names
Selenite, Selenium Dioxide, Selenized Yeast, Selenomethionine

Principal Proposed Uses
Cancer Prevention

Other Proposed Uses
Diabetic Neuropathy, Acne, AIDS, Asthma, Cataracts, Cervical Dysplasia, Heart Disease, Multiple Sclerosis, Rheumatoid Arthritis, Anxiety, Gout, Male Infertility, Osteoarthritis, Psoriasis, Ulcers

Selenium is a trace mineral that our bodies use to produce *glutathione peroxidase,* an enzyme that serves as a natural antioxidant. Glutathione peroxidase works with vitamin E to protect cell membranes from damage caused by dangerous, naturally occurring substances known as free radicals.

You may have heard that China has very low rates of colon cancer, presumably because of the nation's low-fat diet. However, in some parts of China where the soil is depleted of selenium, the incidence of various types of cancer is much higher than in the rest of the country. This fact has given rise to a theory that selenium deficiency is a common cause of cancer, and that selenium supplements can reduce this risk.

As we will see, there is some real evidence that selenium supplements can provide some protection against several types of cancer. This "chemopreventive" effect isn't fully understood. It might be due to the protective effects of the antioxidant glutathione peroxidase, but other explanations have also been suggested.[1,2]

Requirements/Sources

The U.S. Recommended Dietary Allowance for selenium is as follows

- Infants under 6 months, 10 mcg
    6 to 12 months, 15 mcg
- Children 1 to 6 years, 20 mcg
    7 to 10 years, 30 mcg
- Males 11 to 14 years, 40 mcg
    15 to 18 years, 50 mcg
    19 years and older, 70 mcg
- Females 11 to 14 years, 45 mcg
    15 to 18 years, 50 mcg
    19 years and older, 55 mcg
- Pregnant women, 65 mcg
- Nursing women, 75 mcg

Studies suggest that many people in developed countries do not get enough selenium in their diets.[3]

Foods containing significant amounts of selenium include wheat germ, nuts (particularly Brazil nuts), oats, whole-wheat bread, bran, red Swiss chard, brown rice, turnips, garlic, barley, and orange juice.

However, even these foods won't give you an adequate intake if the soil they were grown in was poor in selenium. Unfortunately, most of us have no way of knowing what kind of soil our food was grown in, so supplements may be a good idea.

The two general types of selenium supplements available to consumers are organic and inorganic. These terms have a very specific chemical meaning and have nothing to do with "organic" foods. In chemistry, organic means a substance's chemical structure includes carbon. Inorganic chemicals have no carbon atoms.

The inorganic form of selenium, selenite, is essentially selenium atoms bound to oxygen. Some research suggests that selenite is harder for the body to absorb than organic forms of selenium, such as selenomethionine (selenium bound to methionine, an essential amino acid) or high-selenium yeast (which contains selenomethionine).[4,5] However, other research on both animals and humans suggests that selenite supplements are almost as good as organic forms of selenium.[6,7]

Therapeutic Dosages

In controlled trials of selenium, a typical dosage was 100 to 200 mcg daily, in the same ballpark as nutritional doses.

Therapeutic Uses

Impressive evidence indicates that supplemental selenium may help prevent cancer.[8–13] One study suggests that selenium might help diabetic neuropathy.[14] Additionally, based on what science knows about antioxidants in general, selenium has been proposed as a preventive measure or treatment for acne, AIDS, asthma, cataracts, cervical dysplasia, heart disease, multiple sclerosis, and rheumatoid arthritis. Besides the antioxidant rationale, people with these conditions often have lower-than-normal tissue levels of selenium. This suggests that selenium supplements might be a good treatment for these conditions. However, it is definitely not proof, and in the case of rheumatoid arthritis at least, there's some evidence that selenium supplements *don't* help.[15]

Selenium has also been recommended for many other conditions, including anxiety, gout, male infertility, osteoarthritis, psoriasis, and ulcers, but there is no real evidence as yet that it really works.

What Is the Scientific Evidence for Selenium?

Cancer Prevention

A large body of evidence has found that increased intake of selenium is tied to a reduced risk of cancer. The most important blind study on selenium and cancer was a double-blind intervention trial conducted by researchers at the University of Arizona Cancer Center. In this trial, which began in 1983, 1,312 individuals were divided into two groups. One group received 200 mcg of yeast-based selenium daily; the other received placebo.[16] The researchers were trying to determine whether selenium could lower the incidence of skin cancers.

Although they found no benefit for skin cancer, they saw dramatic declines in the incidence of several other cancers in the selenium group. For ethical reasons, researchers felt compelled to stop the study after several years and allow all participants to take selenium.

When all the results were tabulated, it became clear that the selenium-treated group developed almost 66% fewer prostate cancers, 50% fewer colorectal cancers, and about 40% fewer lung cancers as compared with the placebo group. (All these results were statistically significant.) Selenium-treated subjects also experienced a statistically significant (17%) decrease in overall mortality, a greater than 50% decrease in lung cancer deaths, and nearly a 50% decrease in total cancer deaths.

Further evidence for the anticancer benefits of selenium comes from large-scale Chinese studies showing that giving selenium supplements to people who live in selenium-deficient areas reduces the incidence of cancer.[17]

Also, observational studies have indicated that cancer deaths rise when dietary intake of selenium is low.[18,19]

The results of animal studies corroborate these results. One recent animal study examined whether two experimental organic forms of selenium would protect laboratory rats against chemically induced cancer of the tongue.[20] Rats were given one of three treatments: 5 parts per million of selenium in their drinking water, 15 parts per million of selenium, or placebo. The study was blinded so that the researchers wouldn't know until later which rats received which treatment. Whereas 47% of the rats in the placebo group developed tongue tumors, none of the rats that were given the higher selenium dosage developed tumors.

Another study examined whether selenium supplements could stop the spread (metastasis) of cancer in mice. In this study, a modest dosage of supplemental selenium reduced metastasis by 57%.[21] Even more significant was the decrease in the number of tumors that had spread to the lungs: mice in the control group had an average of 53 tumors each, whereas mice fed supplemental selenium had an average of one lung tumor.

Putting all this information together, it definitely appears that selenium can help reduce the risk of developing cancer.

Safety Issues

Selenium is safe when taken at the recommended dosages. However, very high selenium dosages, above 850 mcg daily, are known to cause selenium toxicity. Signs of selenium toxicity include depression, nervousness, emotional instability, nausea, vomiting, and in some cases loss of hair and fingernails.

⚠ Interactions You Should Know About

If you are taking **antacids**, you may need extra selenium.

SOY

Supplement Forms/Alternate Names
Hydrolyzed Soy Protein, Soy Protein, Soy Protein Extract
Principal Proposed Uses
High Cholesterol
Other Proposed Uses
Menopausal Symptoms, Cancer Prevention

The soybean has been prized for centuries in Asia as a nutritious, high-protein food with myriad uses, and today it's popular in the United States not only in Asian food but also as a cholesterol-free meat and dairy substitute in traditional American foods. Soy burgers, soy yogurt, tofu hot dogs, and tofu cheese can be found in a growing number of grocery stores alongside the traditional white blocks of tofu.

Soybeans contain chemicals that are similar to estrogen. These are probably the active ingredient in soy, although we don't know for sure. They are described in more detail in the chapter on isoflavones. Soy appears to reduce blood cholesterol levels, and the U.S. Food and Drug Administration has authorized allowing foods containing soy to carry a "heart-healthy" label.

Most likely, it is the isoflavone part of soy that provides most of its benefits.

Sources

If you like Japanese, Chinese, Thai, or Vietnamese food, it's easy to get a healthy dose of soy. Tofu is one of the world's most versatile foods. It can be stir-fried, steamed, or added to soup. You can also mash a cake of tofu and use it in place of ricotta cheese in your lasagna. If you don't like tofu, there are many other soy products to try: plain soybeans, soy cheese, soy burgers, soy milk, or tempeh. Or you can use a soy supplement instead.

Dosages

The FDA suggests a daily intake of 25 g of soy protein to reduce cholesterol. This amount is typically found in about 2½ cups of soy milk or ½ pound of tofu. Studies have used dosages of up to 40 g daily. If you prefer to use isolated soy isoflavones, 62 mg daily appears to be enough to reduce cholesterol.[1]

Therapeutic Uses

According to the combined evidence of 38 controlled studies, soy can reduce blood cholesterol levels and improve the ratio of LDL ("bad") versus HDL ("good") cholesterol.[2] With an average dosage of 47 g daily, total cholesterol falls by about 9%, LDL cholesterol by 13%, and triglycerides by 10%. Soy's effects on HDL cholesterol itself are less impressive.

Soy also seems to reduce the common menopausal symptom known as "hot flashes."[3] Unlike estrogen, soy appears to reduce the risk of uterine cancer.[4] Its effect on breast cancer is not as well established, but there are reasons to believe that soy can help reduce breast cancer risk as well.[5,6,7] Although we don't know for sure, soy may do this by reducing levels of estrogen in the blood.[8,9] Soy may also help prevent prostate and colon cancer.[10,11,12]

What Is the Scientific Evidence for Soy?

High Cholesterol

In 1995, a review of 38 controlled studies on soy and heart disease concluded that soy is effective at reducing total cholesterol, LDL ("bad") cholesterol, and triglycerides.[13] It appears that the isoflavones in soy are the active ingredient.[14]

Another double-blind study (not part of the review mentioned previously), which involved 66 older women, found improvements in HDL ("good") cholesterol as well.[15] The women were divided into three groups. The first group received 40 g of skim milk protein daily. The second group was given the same amount of soy protein, and the third received

40 g of soy protein with extra soy isoflavones. Compared with the skim milk (placebo) group, both soy groups showed significant improvements in both total cholesterol and HDL cholesterol.

One benefit from eating soy is that, unlike most other sources of protein, it contains no fat. However, soy produces benefits above and beyond substituting for less healthful forms of protein.[16]

Menopausal Symptoms ("Hot Flashes")

Soy seems to relieve "hot flashes," a common symptom of menopause. A double-blind placebo-controlled study involving 104 women found that soy provided significant relief compared to placebo (milk protein). After 3 weeks, the women taking daily doses of 60 g of soy protein were having 26% fewer hot flashes.[17] By week 12, the reduction was 45%. Women taking placebo also experienced a big improvement by week 12 (30% fewer hot flashes), but soy gave significantly better results.

It is thought that the isoflavones in soy are responsible for these effects.[18]

Safety Issues

As a food that has been eaten for centuries, soy is believed to be quite safe. However, the isoflavones in soy could conceivably have some potentially harmful hormonal effects in certain specific situations. There is some evidence that although soy generally seems to reduce the risk of breast cancer, it also may cause some influences in the opposite direction.[19] For this and other reasons, we don't know if high doses of soy are safe for women who have already had breast cancer (for more information, see the chapter on isoflavones). Soy may also interact with hormone medications. Finally, there are also concerns that intensive use of soy products by pregnant women could exert a hormonal effect that impacts unborn fetuses.[20,21]

In addition, soy may impair thyroid function or reduce absorption of thyroid medication, at least in children.[22,23,24] For this reason, individuals with impaired thyroid function should use soy with caution.

⚠ Interactions You Should Know About

If you are taking

- **Zinc**, **iron**, or **calcium** supplements: It may be best to eat soy at a different time of day to avoid absorption problems.[25,26,27]
- **Oral contraceptives**: It is possible that soy might interfere with their effects.
- **Thyroid hormone**: It is possible that soy might impair absorption of thyroid medication, at least in children.

TAURINE

Supplement Forms/Alternate Names
L-Taurine

Principal Proposed Uses
Congestive Heart Failure, Viral Hepatitis

Other Proposed Uses
Alcoholism, Cataracts, Diabetes, Epilepsy, Gallbladder Disease, Hypertension (High Blood Pressure), Multiple Sclerosis, Psoriasis, Stroke

Taurine is an amino acid, one of the building blocks of proteins. Found in the nervous system and muscles, taurine is one of the most abundant amino acids in the body. It is thought to help regulate heartbeat, maintain cell membranes, and affect the release of neurotransmitters (chemicals that carry signals between nerve cells) in the brain.

Taurine's best-established use is to treat congestive heart failure (CHF), a condition in which the heart muscle progressively weakens. It may also be useful for hepatitis.

Warning: Please keep in mind that CHF is too serious for self-treatment. If you're interested in trying taurine or any other supplement for CHF, you should first consult your doctor.

Sources

There is no dietary requirement for taurine, since the body can make it out of vitamin B_6 and the amino acids methionine and cysteine. Deficiencies occasionally occur in vegetarians, whose diets may not provide the building blocks for making taurine.

People with diabetes have lower-than-average blood levels of taurine, but whether this means they should take extra taurine is unclear.

Meat, poultry, eggs, dairy products, and fish are good sources of taurine. Legumes and nuts don't contain taurine, but they do contain methionine and cysteine.

Therapeutic Dosages

A typical therapeutic dosage of taurine is 2 g 3 times daily.

Therapeutic Uses

Preliminary evidence suggests that taurine might be helpful in congestive heart failure, a condition in which the heart has trouble pumping blood, which leads to fluid accumulating in the legs and lungs.[1]

There is also some evidence that taurine may be helpful for acute viral hepatitis.[2]

Taurine has additionally been proposed as a treatment for numerous other conditions, including alcoholism, cataracts, diabetes, epilepsy, gallbladder disease, hypertension, multiple sclerosis, psoriasis, and stroke, but the evidence for these uses is weak and, in some cases, contradictory.[3–7] Taurine is also sometimes combined in an "amino acid cocktail" with other amino acids for treatment of attention deficit disorder, but there is no evidence as yet that it works for this purpose.

What Is the Scientific Evidence for Taurine?

Congestive Heart Failure

Several studies (primarily by one researcher) suggest that taurine may be useful for congestive heart failure (CHF).

For example, in one double-blind trial, 58 people with CHF took either placebo or 2 g of taurine 3 times daily for 4 weeks.[8] Then the groups were switched. During taurine treatment, the study participants showed highly significant improvement in breathlessness, heart palpitations, fluid buildup, and heart x ray, as well as standard scales of heart failure severity. Animal research as well as small, blinded or open studies in humans have also found positive effects.[9–13] Interestingly, one very small study compared taurine with another supplement commonly used for congestive heart failure, coenzyme Q_{10}. The results suggest that taurine is more effective.[14] (For more information see Coenzyme Q_{10}.)

Viral Hepatitis

There are several viruses that can cause acute hepatitis, a disabling and sometimes dangerous infection of the liver. The most common are hepatitis A and B, although there are others (with such imaginative names as C and D).

One double-blind study suggests that taurine supplements might be useful for acute viral hepatitis. In this double-blind placebo-controlled study, 63 people with hepatitis were given either 12 g of taurine daily or placebo.[15] (The report does not state what type of viral hepatitis they had.) According to blood tests, the taurine group experienced significant improvements in liver function as compared to the placebo group.

Acute hepatitis can also develop into a long-lasting or permanent condition known as chronic hepatitis. One small double-blind study suggests that taurine does not help chronic hepatitis.[16] For this purpose, the herb milk thistle may be better.

Safety Issues

As an amino acid found in food, taurine is thought to be quite safe. However, maximum safe dosages of taurine supplements for children, pregnant or nursing women, or those with severe liver or kidney disease have not been determined.

As with any supplement taken in multigram doses, it is important to purchase a reputable product, because a contaminant present even in small percentages could add up to a real problem.

TMG (TRIMETHYLGLYCINE)

Supplement Forms/Alternate Names
Betaine (Similar to betaine hydrochloride, but not identical)

Principal Proposed Uses
There are no documented uses for TMG.

Other Proposed Uses
Reducing Homocysteine Levels, Liver Protection, Substitute for SAMe, Enhancing Athletic Performance

---

TMG (trimethylglycine) has been available for decades. Recently, it has drawn attention as a possible treatment for elevated homocysteine levels.

Homocysteine is a naturally occurring chemical that may be as harmful to blood vessels as cholesterol. Folate and vitamin B_6 destroy homocysteine by "methylating" it—attaching one carbon atom and three hydrogen atoms to it. This makes homocysteine harmless. Recent studies have found that vitamin B_6 and folate can help prevent heart disease, apparently by lowering homocysteine levels in the blood.

After this discovery, great interest developed in other substances that can methylate homocysteine. Chemicals of this type are called "methylating agents." SAMe (S-adenosylmethionine) is one; TMG is another. However, research into this subject is still in its infancy.

After TMG has done its work on homocysteine, it is turned into another substance, dimethylglycine (DMG). In Russia, DMG is used extensively as an athletic performance enhancer; however, TMG is cheaper and may have the same effects (if any).

Sources

TMG is not required in the diet because the body can manufacture it from other nutrients. Grains, nuts, seeds, and meats contain small amounts of TMG. However, most TMG in food is destroyed during cooking or processing, so food isn't a reliable way to get a therapeutic dosage.

Some manufacturers will tell you that DMG is identical to TMG, but this isn't true. DMG is not a methylating agent, so it can't have any effect on homocysteine.

Therapeutic Dosages

There hasn't been enough research to establish the optimal therapeutic dosage of TMG. One manufacturer recommends using between 375 and 1,000 mg daily.

Therapeutic Uses

One small study suggests that TMG may lower homocysteine levels,[1] which might be helpful for those with atherosclerosis.

TMG may also help protect the liver against the effects of alcohol, perhaps by stimulating the formation of SAMe.[2,3,4] Additionally, it may be useful for other purposes for which SAMe is used, although this has not been proven.

DMG (the substance TMG changes into in the body) has been extensively used as a performance enhancer by Russian athletes, and has recently become popular among American athletes. However, one small study suggests that it does not work.[5]

Safety Issues

TMG appears to be safe. However, the maximum safe dosages for young children, pregnant or nursing mothers, or those with severe liver or kidney disease have not been established.

TYROSINE

Supplement Forms/Alternate Names
L-Tyrosine
Principal Proposed Uses
There are no well-documented uses for tyrosine.
Other Proposed Uses
Sleep Deprivation, Attention Deficit Disorder, Depression

Tyrosine is an amino acid found in meat proteins. Your body uses it as a starting material to make several neurotransmitters (chemicals that help the brain and nervous system function). Based on this fact, tyrosine has been proposed as a treatment for various conditions in which mental function is impaired or slowed down, such as sleep deprivation and depression. It has also been tried for attention deficit disorder (ADD).

Sources

Your body makes tyrosine from another common amino acid, *phenylalanine*, so deficiencies are rare; however, they can occur in certain forms of severe kidney disease as well as in phenylketonuria (PKU), a metabolic disorder that requires complete avoidance of phenylalanine. (For more information, see the chapter on phenylalanine.)

Good sources of tyrosine include dairy products, meats, fish, and beans.

Therapeutic Dosages

The typical recommended dosage of tyrosine is 7 to 30 g daily.

Therapeutic Uses

According to very preliminary evidence, tyrosine supplements may help fight fatigue and increase alertness in people who are deprived of sleep.[1]

Tyrosine may also provide some temporary benefit for attention deficit disorder, but the benefits appear to wear off in a couple of weeks.[2,3,4] Tyrosine is said to work better for this purpose when it is combined in an "amino acid cocktail" along with gamma-aminobutyric acid (GABA), phenylalanine, and glutamine; however, there is no scientific evidence to support this use.

Although one extremely tiny study found tyrosine helpful for depression,[5] a recent larger study found it not effective.[6]

What Is the Scientific Evidence for Tyrosine?

Sleep Deprivation

A placebo-controlled study that enrolled 20 U.S. Marines suggests that tyrosine can improve alertness during periods of sleep deprivation. In this study, the participants were deprived of sleep for a night and then tested frequently for their alertness throughout the day as they worked. Compared to placebo, 10 to 15 g of tyrosine given twice daily seemed to provide a "pick-up" for about 2 hours.[7]

Depression

A study that enrolled nine individuals is widely quoted as evidence that tyrosine can help depression.[8] However, a recent double-blind placebo-controlled study of 65 people with depression found *no* benefit.[9]

Safety Issues

Tyrosine seems to be generally safe, though at high dosages some people have reported nausea, diarrhea, vomiting, or nervousness. As with any other supplement taken in multigram doses, it is important to use a high-quality product; even a very small percentage of contaminant in the product might add up to a dangerous amount.

Maximum safe dosages for young children, women who are pregnant or nursing, or those with severe liver or kidney disease have not been established.

VANADIUM

Supplement Forms/Alternate Names
Vanadate, Vanadyl Sulfate
Principal Proposed Uses
There are no well-documented uses for vanadium, and there are serious safety concerns regarding vanadium use.
Other Proposed Uses
Diabetes, Bodybuilding, Osteoporosis

Vanadium, a mineral, is named after the Scandinavian goddess of beauty, youth, and luster. Taking vanadium will not make you beautiful, youthful, and lustrous, but evidence from animal studies suggests it may be an essential micronutrient. That is, your body may need it, but in very low doses.

Based on promising animal studies, high doses of vanadium have been tested as an aid to controlling blood sugar levels in people with diabetes. Like chromium, another trace mineral used in diabetes, vanadium has also been recommended as an aid in bodybuilding. However, animal studies suggest that taking high doses of vanadium can be harmful.

Requirements/Sources

We don't know exactly how much vanadium people require, but estimates range from 10 to 30 mcg daily. (To realize how tiny this amount is, consider that it's about *one millionth* of the amount of calcium you need.) Human deficiencies have not been reported, but goats fed a low-vanadium diet have developed birth defects.[1]

Vanadium is found in very small amounts in a wide variety of foods, including breakfast cereals, canned fruit juices, wine, beer, buckwheat, parsley, soy, oats, olive oil, sunflower seeds, corn, green beans, peanut oil, carrots, cabbage, and garlic. The average daily American diet provides between 10 and 60 mcg of vanadium.[2]

Therapeutic Dosages

In various studies, vanadium has been used at doses thousands of times higher than is present in the diet, as high as 125 mg per day. However, there are serious safety concerns about taking vanadium at such high doses (see Safety Issues). We do not recommend exceeding the nutritional dose of 10 to 30 mcg daily.

Therapeutic Uses

Vanadium has been proposed as a treatment for diabetes, based on promising studies in animals and a few small human trials.[3,4]

Vanadium is also sometimes used by bodybuilders, but there is no evidence that it is effective.[5]

Because studies in mice have found that vanadium is deposited in bone,[6] some practitioners of nutritional medicine have suggested that it may be helpful for osteoporosis. However, since many toxic metals also accumulate in the bones without strengthening them, this doesn't prove that vanadium is good for bones.

What Is the Scientific Evidence for Vanadium?

Diabetes

Studies in rats with and without diabetes suggest that vanadium may have an insulin-like effect, reducing blood sugar levels.[7–17] Based on these findings, preliminary studies involving human subjects have been conducted, with promising results.[18–21] However, they were all too small to be taken as definitive proof. More research is needed to definitely establish whether vanadium is effective (not to mention safe) for the treatment of diabetes.

Bodybuilding

A double-blind placebo-controlled study involving 31 weight-trained athletes found *no* benefit at a dosage more than 1,000 times the nutritional dose.[22]

Safety Issues

Studies in humans and animals suggest that vanadium can cause toxic effects and might accumulate in the body if taken to excess.[23–26] Based on these results, high dosages of vanadium can't be considered safe for human use. If you wish to take it, stick to the 10 to 30 mcg a day mentioned earlier.

VINPOCETINE

Supplement Forms/Alternate Names
Periwinkle

Principal Proposed Uses
Alzheimer's Disease, Other Forms of Dementia, Ordinary Age-Related Memory Loss

Vinpocetine (vin-PO-se-teen) is a chemical derived from vincamine, a constituent found in the leaves of common periwinkle (*Vinca minor* L.) as well as the seeds of various African plants. It is used as a treatment for memory loss and mental impairment.

Developed in Hungary over 20 years ago, vinpocetine is sold in Europe as a drug under the name Cavinton. In the United States it is available as a "dietary supplement," although the substance probably doesn't fit that category by any rational definition. Vinpocetine doesn't exist to any significant extent in nature. Producing it requires significant chemical work performed in the laboratory.

What Is the Scientific Evidence for Vinpocetine?

A significant level of evidence supports the idea that vinpocetine can enhance memory and mental function, especially in those with Alzheimer's disease and related conditions. It may also be helpful for those with ordinary age-related memory loss, although this has not been proven.

One 3-month double-blind placebo-controlled study followed 84 individuals with age-related mental impairment.[1] According to several standard rating scales, the severity of the illness improved by a statistically significant margin in the treatment group as compared to the placebo group. Similarly positive results have been seen in many other studies,[2] although at least one study did not find benefit.[3]

We don't know how vinpocetine works, although there are numerous theories. There is some evidence that vinpocetine can safeguard brain cells against damage caused by lack of oxygen.[4] However, whether this effect really has anything to do with its effects on mental function remains unclear.

Dosage

Vinpocetine is available in 10-mg capsules, usually taken 3 times per day. This supplement is probably best taken with meals, as it is better absorbed that way.[5] We recommend that it be used only on physician advice.

Safety Issues

No serious side effects have been reported in any of the clinical trials. However, there are some concerns that vinpocetine might impair the effectiveness of Coumadin (warfarin).[6] Safety in pregnant women or those with severe liver or kidney disease has not been established.

VITAMIN A

Supplement Forms/Alternate Names
Retinol

Principal Proposed Uses
Viral Infections in Children in Developing Countries

Other Proposed Uses
Diabetes

Skin Disorders: Acne, Psoriasis

Menorrhagia (Heavy Menstruation), AIDS, Down's Syndrome, Ear Infections, Eating Disorders, Glaucoma, Gout, Impaired Night Vision, Kidney Stones, Lupus, Multiple Sclerosis, Ulcerative Colitis, Ulcers, Crohn's Disease

Note: Beta-carotene is sometimes used interchangeably with vitamin A, because the body can turn beta-carotene into vitamin A.

Vitamin A is a fat-soluble antioxidant that protects your cells against damaging free radicals and plays other vital roles in the body. However, it is potentially more dangerous than most other vitamins because it can build up to toxic levels, causing liver damage and birth defects. Because of this risk, vitamin A supplements have few therapeutic uses.

In general, beta-carotene supplements taken at nutritional doses are a safer way to get the vitamin A you need. Sometimes called "provitamin A," beta-carotene is transformed into vitamin A as your body needs it, and presents much less risk of toxicity.

Requirements/Sources

Vitamin A is an essential nutrient—meaning you must get it in the diet. The U.S. Recommended Dietary Allowance is as follows

- Infants under 1 year, 1,250 IU; 375 mcg (or retinol equivalent, RE)
- Children 1 to 3 years, 1,333 IU; 400 mcg
  4 to 6 years, 1,667 IU; 500 mcg
  7 to 10 years, 2,333 IU; 700 mcg

- Males 11 years and older, 3,333 IU; 1,000 mcg
- Females 11 years and older, 2,667 IU; 800 mcg
- Pregnant women, 2,667 IU; 800 mcg
- Nursing women, 4,000 to 4,338 IU; 1,200 to 1,300 mcg

These amounts can be obtained safely by taking beta-carotene instead of vitamin A. The proper dose may be calculated by keeping in mind that 1 IU of beta-carotene is equivalent to 1 IU of vitamin A; 1 mg of beta-carotene is equivalent to 500 mcg of vitamin A.

Warning: Pregnant women should not take vitamin A supplements. Instead they should take beta-carotene.

We get vitamin A from many foods, in the form of either vitamin A or beta-carotene. Liver and dairy products are excellent sources of vitamin A. Carrots, apricots, collard greens, kale, sweet potatoes, parsley, and spinach are good sources as well.

Deficiency in vitamin A is common in developing countries.[1] In the developed world, deficiency is relatively rare, except among teenagers and those in lower socioeconomic groups. Also, the older cholesterol-lowering drugs cholestyramine and colestipol can reduce vitamin A levels.[2]

Therapeutic Dosages

Doses of vitamin A above the basic nutritional requirement are not recommended.

Therapeutic Uses

There is some evidence that vitamin A supplements reduce deaths from measles and other causes among children in developing countries,[3] presumably because they correct a deficiency in the children's diets. This doesn't mean that vitamin A supplements above and beyond the basic nutritional requirement are a useful treatment for measles or any other childhood disease.

Vitamin A may be helpful for diabetes. However, there are concerns that people with diabetes may be especially vulnerable to liver damage from excessive amounts of vitamin A (see Safety Issues). Therefore, if you have diabetes, you should take vitamin A only on the advice of a physician.

Vitamin A has been used in the past for a variety of skin diseases such as acne and psoriasis, but since you need to use large amounts (which could cause toxicity) to achieve benefits, standard medications are safer. High-dose vitamin A may also be helpful for menorrhagia (heavy menstruation),[4] but again it is not safe.

In addition, vitamin A has been proposed as a treatment for a wide variety of other conditions, some of them quite serious, including AIDS, Down's syndrome, ear infections, eating disorders, glaucoma, gout, impaired night vision, kidney stones, lupus, multiple sclerosis, ulcerative colitis, and ulcers. There is little to no evidence that it is effective for any of these conditions. One study suggests that vitamin A is not effective for Crohn's disease.[5]

What Is the Scientific Evidence for Vitamin A?

Viral Infections (in Children Living in Developing Countries)
Vitamin A has been tried as a treatment for various viral infections, including measles, respiratory syncytial virus (RSV, a common childhood viral disease of the respiratory tract), chicken pox, and AIDS.

Most of the research on vitamin A has concentrated on children in developing countries. A review article examining 12 studies suggested that vitamin A supplements can protect such children from dying and should be used more widely.[6]

Success with measles led researchers to study its use in respiratory syncytial virus.[7,8] However, the results were not impressive.

Diabetes
According to many[9,10] but not all[11,12] studies, people with diabetes tend to be deficient in vitamin A.

An observational study suggests that vitamin A supplements may improve blood sugar control in people with diabetes.[13] However, due to safety concerns, they should not supplement with vitamin A except under medical supervision (see Safety Issues).

Skin Disorders

Vitamin A has been tried for various skin disorders, including acne, psoriasis, rosacea, seborrhea, and eczema.[14–17] However, the benefits have not been great, and generally vitamin A has to be taken in potentially toxic dosages to produce good effects.

Menorrhagia (Heavy Menstruation)

One study suggests that women with heavy menstrual bleeding can benefit from taking 25,000 IU daily of vitamin A.[18] But vitamin A cannot be recommended as an ongoing treatment for menorrhagia, since women who menstruate can become pregnant, and even low doses of supplemental vitamin A may cause birth defects.

Crohn's Disease

According to a double-blind study of 86 people with Crohn's disease, vitamin A does not help prevent flare-ups.[19]

Safety Issues

Dosages of vitamin A above 50,000 IU per day taken for several years can cause liver injury, bone problems, fatigue, hair loss, headaches, and dry skin. If you already have liver disease, check with your doctor before taking vitamin A supplements, because even small doses may be harmful for you. Also, it is thought that people with diabetes may have trouble releasing vitamin A stored in the liver. This may mean that they are at greater risk for vitamin A toxicity. For different reasons, individuals who consume too much alcohol may also be at higher risk of vitamin A toxicity.[20] In addition, excessive intake of vitamin A may increase the risk of osteoporosis.[21]

Women should avoid supplementing with vitamin A during pregnancy, because at toxic levels it may increase the risk of birth defects.

Warning: Be sure to store vitamin A supplements where children cannot reach them!

⚠ Interactions You Should Know About

If you are taking

- The older cholesterol-lowering drugs **cholestyramine** or **colestipol**: You may need more vitamin A (preferably as beta-carotene).
- **Isotretinoin (Accutane):** Don't take vitamin A as they might enhance each other's toxicity.

VITAMIN B₁

Supplement Forms/Alternate Names
Thiamin

Principal Proposed Uses
Congestive Heart Failure, Nutritional Support

Other Proposed Uses
Alzheimer's Disease, Epilepsy, Canker Sores, Fibromyalgia

Vitamin B₁, also called thiamin, was the first B vitamin ever discovered. Your body uses it to process fats, carbohydrates, and proteins. Every cell in your body needs thiamin to make adenosine triphosphate, or ATP, the body's main energy-carrying molecule. The heart, in particular, has considerable need for thiamin in order to keep up its constant work.

Severe deficiency results in beriberi, a disease common among sailors through the nineteenth century, but rare today. Beriberi is still seen, however, in developing countries as well as in alcoholics and people with diseases that significantly impair the body's ability to absorb vitamin B₁. Many of the principal symptoms of beriberi relate to impaired heart function.

Requirements/Sources

Your need for vitamin B₁ varies with age. The U.S. Recommended Dietary Allowance is as follows

- Infants under 6 months, 0.3 mg
  6 months to 1 year, 0.4 mg
- Children 1 to 3 years, 0.7 mg
  4 to 6 years, 0.9 mg
  7 to 10 years, 1.0 mg
- Males 11 to 14 years, 1.3 mg
  15 to 50 years, 1.5 mg
  51 years and older, 1.2 mg
- Females 11 to 50 years, 1.1 mg
  51 years and older, 1.0 mg
- Pregnant women, 1.5 mg
- Nursing women, 1.6 mg

Alcoholism, congestive heart failure, Crohn's disease, anorexia, kidney dialysis, folate deficiency, and multiple sclerosis may all lead to a vitamin B_1 deficiency, and people with these conditions should consider taking B_1 supplements. Certain foods may impair your body's absorption of B_1 as well, including fish, shrimp, clams, mussels, and the herb horsetail.

Brewer's and nutritional yeast are the richest sources of B_1. Peas, beans, nuts, seeds, and whole grains also provide fairly good amounts.

Therapeutic Dosages

Very high dosages of B_1—up to 8 g daily—have been recommended for a variety of conditions.

Since the B vitamins tend to work together, many nutritional experts recommend taking B_1 with other B vitamins in the form of a B-complex supplement.

Therapeutic Uses

Congestive heart failure (CHF) is a condition in which the pumping ability of the heart declines, and fluid begins to accumulate in the lungs and legs. Standard treatment for CHF includes strong "water pills" called loop diuretics. These diuretics, however, deplete the body of B_1.[1] Since the heart depends on vitamin B_1 for its proper function, this is potentially quite worrisome. There is some evidence that supplementation with B$_1$ can improve symptoms.[2,3]

Individuals with alcoholism, Crohn's disease, anorexia, or multiple sclerosis may also benefit from thiamin supplementation as part of general nutritional support.

In addition, weak and contradictory evidence suggests that vitamin B$_1$ may be helpful for Alzheimer's disease.[4-8] Vitamin B$_1$ has also been proposed as a treatment for epilepsy, canker sores, and fibromyalgia, but the evidence for these uses is too preliminary to cite.

What Is the Scientific Evidence for Vitamin B$_1$?

Congestive Heart Failure

Evidence suggests that individuals with congestive heart failure are commonly deficient in vitamin B$_1$, due to their use of loop diuretics.[9] A small double-blind study found that intravenous administration of thiamin could improve heart function in individuals with CHF.[10] Similar results were seen in an earlier uncontrolled study.[11]

Safety Issues

Vitamin B$_1$ appears to be quite safe even when taken in very high doses.

⚠ Interactions You Should Know About

If you are taking **loop diuretics** (e.g., **furosemide [Lasix]**), you may need extra vitamin B$_1$.[12,13,14]

VITAMIN B$_2$

Supplement Forms/Alternate Names

Riboflavin, Riboflavin-5-Phosphate

Principal Proposed Uses

There are no well-documented uses for vitamin B$_2$.

Other Proposed Uses

Migraine Headaches, Cataracts, Sickle-Cell Anemia, Athletic Performance

---

Riboflavin, also known as vitamin B$_2$, is an essential nutrient required for life. This vitamin works with two enzymes critical to the body's production of adenosine triphosphate, or ATP, its main energy source. Vitamin B$_2$ is also used to process amino acids and fats, and to activate vitamin B$_6$ and folate.

Preliminary evidence suggests that riboflavin supplements may offer benefits for two illnesses: migraine headaches and cataracts.

Requirements/Sources

The U.S. Recommended Dietary Allowance for riboflavin is as follows

- Infants under 6 months, 0.4 mg
  6 to 12 months, 0.5 mg
- Children 1 to 3 years, 0.8 mg
  4 to 6 years, 1.1 mg
  7 to 10 years, 1.2 mg
- Males 11 to 14 years, 1.5 mg
  15 to 18 years, 1.8 mg
  19 to 50 years, 1.7 mg
  51 years and older, 1.4 mg
- Females, 11 to 50 years, 1.3 mg
  51 years and older, 1.2 mg
- Pregnant women, 1.6 mg
- Nursing women, 1.7 to 1.8 mg

Riboflavin is found in organ meats (such as liver, kidney, and heart) and in many vegetables, nuts, legumes, and leafy greens. The richest sources are torula (nutritional) yeast, brewer's yeast, and calf liver. Almonds, wheat germ, wild rice, and mushrooms are good sources as well.

Although serious riboflavin deficiencies are rare, slightly low levels can occur in children, the elderly, and those in poverty.[1-4]

Therapeutic Dosages

For migraine headaches, the typical recommended dosage of riboflavin is much higher than nutritional needs: 400 mg daily. For cataract prevention, riboflavin may be taken at the nutritional dosages described. Since the B vitamins tend to work together, many nutritional experts recommend taking B_2 with other B vitamins, perhaps in the form of a B-complex supplement.

Therapeutic Uses

There are no well-documented uses of riboflavin. However, preliminary evidence suggests that riboflavin supplements taken at high dosages may reduce the frequency of migraine headaches.[5]

One very large study suggests that riboflavin at nutritional doses may be helpful for cataracts, but in this study it was combined with another B vitamin, niacin or vitamin B_3, so it's hard to say which vitamin was responsible for the effect.[6]

Riboflavin has also been proposed as a treatment for sickle-cell anemia[7] and as a performance enhancer for athletes, but there is no real evidence that it is effective for these uses.

What Is the Scientific Evidence for Vitamin B_2?

Migraine Headaches

According to a 3-month, double-blind, placebo-controlled study of 55 people with migraines, riboflavin can significantly reduce the frequency and duration of migraine attacks.[8] This study found that, when given at least 2 months to work, a daily dose of riboflavin (400 mg) can produce dramatic migraine relief. The majority of the participants experienced a greater than 50% decrease in the number of migraine attacks as well as the total days with headache pain. A larger and longer study is needed to follow up on these results.

Cataracts

Riboflavin supplements may help prevent cataracts, but the evidence isn't yet clear. In a large, double-blind placebo-controlled study, 3,249 people were given either placebo or one of four nutrient combinations (vitamin A/zinc, riboflavin/niacin, vitamin C/molybdenum, or selenium/beta-carotene/vitamin E) for a period of 6 years.[9] Those receiving the niacin/riboflavin supplement showed a significant (44%) reduction in the incidence of cataracts. Strangely, there was a small, but statistically significantly higher incidence of a special type of cataract (called a subcapsular cataract) in the niacin/riboflavin group. However, it is unclear whether the effects seen in this group were due to niacin, riboflavin, or the combination of the two.

Safety Issues

Riboflavin seems to be an extremely safe supplement.

⚠ Interactions You Should Know About

If you are taking **oral contraceptives**, you may need extra riboflavin.

VITAMIN B₃

Supplement Forms/Alternate Names
Inositol Hexaniacinate, Niacin, Niacinamide, Nicotinamide

Principal Proposed Uses
High Cholesterol/Triglycerides (Niacin), Diabetes Prevention and Treatment (Niacinamide), Intermittent Claudication (Inositol Hexaniacinate), Osteoarthritis (Niacinamide), Raynaud's Phenomenon (Inositol Hexaniacinate)

Other Proposed Uses
Bursitis, Cataracts, Pregnancy Support

Vitamin B₃ is required for the proper function of more than 50 enzymes. Without it, your body would not be able to release energy or make fats from carbohydrates. Vitamin B₃ is also used to make sex hormones and other important chemical signal molecules.

Vitamin B₃ comes in two principal forms: niacin (nicotinic acid) and niacinamide (nicotinamide). When taken in low doses for nutritional purposes, they are essentially identical. However, each has its own particular effects when taken in high doses. High-dose niacin is principally used for lowering cholesterol. High-dose niacinamide may be helpful in preventing type 1 (childhood-onset) diabetes and reducing symptoms of osteoarthritis. However, there are concerns regarding liver inflammation when any form of niacin is taken at high dosages.

Additionally, good evidence suggests that a special form of niacin, *inositol hexaniacinate,* can improve walking distance in intermittent claudication. It may also reduce symptoms of Raynaud's phenomenon.

Requirements/Sources

The U.S. Recommended Dietary Allowance for niacin is as follows

- Infants under 6 months, 5 mg
  6 to 12 months, 6 mg

- Children 1 to 3 years, 9 mg
  4 to 6 years, 12 mg
  7 to 10 years, 13 mg
- Males 11 to 14 years, 17 mg
  15 to 18 years, 20 mg
  19 to 50 years, 19 mg
  51 years and older, 15 mg
- Females 11 to 50 years, 15 mg
  51 years and older, 13 mg
- Pregnant women, 17 mg
- Nursing women, 20 mg

Because the body can make niacin from the common amino acid tryptophan, niacin deficiencies are rare in developed countries. However, the antituberculosis drug isoniazid (INH) impairs the conversion of tryptophan to niacin and may produce symptoms of niacin deficiency (see Interactions You Should Know About).[1]

Good food sources of niacin are seeds, yeast, bran, peanuts (especially with skins), wild rice, brown rice, whole wheat, barley, almonds, and peas. Tryptophan is found in protein foods (meat, poultry, dairy products, fish). Turkey and milk are particularly excellent sources of tryptophan.

Therapeutic Dosages

When used as therapy for a specific disease, niacin, niacinamide, and inositol hexaniacinate are taken in dosages much higher than nutritional needs, about 1 to 4 g daily. Because of the risk of liver inflammation at these doses, medical supervision is essential.

For prevention of diabetes in children, the usual dosage of niacinamide is 25 mg per kilogram body weight per day. There are 2.2 pounds in a kilogram, so a 40-pound child would get about 450 mg daily.

Warning: Medical supervision is essential before giving your child long-term niacinamide treatment.

Many people experience an unpleasant flushing sensation and headache when they take niacin. These symptoms can usually be reduced by gradually increasing the dosage over several weeks or by using slow-release niacin. However, slow-release niacin appears to be more likely to cause liver inflammation than other forms. Inositol hexaniacinate may also cause less flushing than plain niacin, and if you take an aspirin along with niacin, the flushing reaction will usually decrease.

Therapeutic Uses

There is no question that niacin (but not niacinamide) can significantly lower total cholesterol and LDL ("bad") cholesterol and raise HDL ("good") cholesterol.[2–6] However, unpleasant flushing reactions and the risk of liver inflammation have kept niacin from being widely used (see Safety Issues).

Intriguing evidence suggests that regular use of niacinamide (but not niacin) may help prevent diabetes in children at special risk of developing it.[7] Risk can be determined by measuring the ratio of antibodies to islet cells (ICA antibody test).

Niacinamide may improve blood sugar control in both children and adults who already have diabetes.[8,9]

According to several good-size, double-blind studies, inositol hexaniacinate may be able to improve walking distance in intermittent claudication (severe leg cramps caused by hardening of the arteries).[10] For other treatments that may help intermittent claudication, see the chapter on carnitine.

Preliminary evidence suggests that inositol hexaniacinate may be able to reduce symptoms of Raynaud's phenomenon as well.[11] This condition includes an extreme response to cold, usually most severely in the hands.

Preliminary evidence suggests that niacinamide may be able to reduce symptoms of osteoarthritis.[12]

Very weak evidence suggests one of the several forms of niacin may be helpful in bursitis,[13] cataracts,[14] and pregnancy.[15]

What Is the Scientific Evidence for Vitamin B₃?

Niacin is one of the best researched of all the vitamins, and the evidence for using it to treat at least one condition—high cholesterol—is strong enough that it has become an accepted mainstream treatment.

High Cholesterol/Triglycerides

Niacin has been used since the 1950s to lower harmful blood lipids (cholesterol, triglycerides, and lipoproteins) and to raise levels of HDL ("good") cholesterol. According to numerous studies, niacin can lower total cholesterol and LDL ("bad") cholesterol by 15 to 25%, lower triglycerides by 2 to 50%, and raise HDL ("good") cholesterol by about 15 to 25%.[16-19] Furthermore, long-term use of niacin has been shown to significantly reduce death rates from cardiovascular disease.[20]

Preventing Diabetes

Exciting evidence from a huge study conducted in New Zealand suggests that niacinamide can prevent high-risk children from developing diabetes.[21] In this study, more than 20,000 children were screened for diabetes risk by measuring ICA antibodies. It turned out that 185 of these children had detectable levels. About 170 of these children were then given niacinamide for 7 years (not all parents agreed to give their children niacinamide or stay in the study for that long). About 10,000 other children were not screened, but they were followed to see whether they developed diabetes.

The results were very impressive. In the group in which children were screened and given niacinamide if they were positive for ICA antibodies, the incidence of diabetes was reduced by as much as 60%.

These findings suggest that niacinamide is a very effective treatment for preventing diabetes. (It also shows that tests for ICA antibodies can very accurately identify children at risk for diabetes.)

At present, an enormous-scale, long-term trial called the European Nicotinamide Diabetes Intervention Trial is being conducted to definitively determine whether regular use of niacinamide can prevent diabetes. Results from the German portion of the study have been released, and they are not positive.[22] However, until the entire study is complete, it is not possible to draw conclusions.

Treating Diabetes

If your child has just developed diabetes, niacinamide may prolong what is called the honeymoon period.[23] This is the interval in which the pancreas can still make some insulin, and insulin needs are low. By giving your child niacinamide, you may be able to buy some time to allow him or her to adjust to a life of insulin injections.

A recent study suggests that niacinamide may also improve blood sugar control in type 2 (adult-onset) diabetes, but it did not use a double-blind design.[24]

Intermittent Claudication

Double-blind studies involving a total of about 400 individuals have found that inositol hexaniacinate can improve walking distance for people with intermittent claudication.[25–28] For example, in one study, 120 individuals were given either placebo or 2 g of inositol hexaniacinate daily. Over a period of 3 months, walking distance improved significantly in the treated group.[29] The effect was roughly comparable to that of L-carnitine.

Osteoarthritis

There is some evidence that niacinamide may provide some benefits for those with osteoarthritis. In a double-blind study, 72 individuals with arthritis were given either 3,000 mg daily of niacinamide (in 5 equal doses) or placebo for 12 weeks.[30] The results showed that treated participants experienced a 29% improvement in symptoms, whereas those given placebo worsened by 10%. However, at this dose, liver inflammation is a concern that must be taken seriously.

Raynaud's Phenomenon

According to one small double-blind study, the inositol hexaniacinate form of niacin may be helpful for Raynaud's phe-

nomenon.[31] The dosage used was 4 g daily, again a dosage
high enough for liver inflammation to be a real possibility.

Safety Issues

When taken at a dosage of more than 100 mg daily, niacin
frequently causes annoying skin flushing, especially in the
face. This reaction may be accompanied by stomach distress,
itching, and headache. In studies, as many as 43% of individuals taking niacin quit because of unpleasant side effects.[32]

A more dangerous effect of niacin is liver inflammation.
Although most commonly seen with slow-release niacin, it
can occur with any type of niacin when taken at a daily dose
of more than 500 mg (usually 3 g or more). Regular blood
tests to evaluate liver function are therefore mandatory when
using high-dose niacin (or niacinamide or inositol hexaniacinate). This side effect almost always goes away when niacin is
stopped.

If you have liver disease, ulcers (presently or in the past),
gout, or diabetes, do not take high-dose niacin except on
medical advice.

Maximum safe dosages for young children and pregnant
or nursing women have not been established.

⚠ Interactions You Should Know About

If you are taking

- **Cholesterol-lowering drugs** in the statin family, or if
  you drink alcohol excessively: Do not take niacin.[33]
- Older cholesterol-lowering drugs such as **cholestyramine** or **colestipol:** You should take niacin at a different time of day to avoid absorption problems.[34]
- **Oral contraceptives:** You may need extra niacin.
- The antituberculosis drug **isoniazid (INH):** You may
  need extra niacin.

VITAMIN B$_6$

Supplement Forms/Alternate Names
Pyridoxal-5-Phosphate, Pyridoxine,Pyridoxine Hydrochloride

Principal Proposed Uses
Heart Disease Prevention, Morning Sickness in Pregnancy, Asthma, PMS

Other Proposed Uses
MSG Sensitivity, Carpal Tunnel Syndrome, Diabetic Neuropathy, Depression, Kidney Stones, Autism (B$_6$ Combined with Magnesium)

Vitamin B$_6$ plays a major role in making proteins, hormones, and neurotransmitters (chemicals that carry signals between nerve cells). Because mild deficiency of vitamin B$_6$ is common, this is one vitamin that is probably worth taking as insurance.

There's good evidence that adequate intake of vitamin B$_6$ can help prevent heart disease and reduce the nausea of morning sickness. This vitamin is also widely recommended for premenstrual syndrome (PMS) and asthma, but there is little evidence that it is effective for either use. When combined with magnesium, vitamin B$_6$ may be helpful for autism.

Requirements/Sources

Vitamin B$_6$ requirements increase with age. The U.S. Recommended Dietary Allowance is as follows

- Infants under 6 months, 0.3 mg
  6 to 12 months, 0.6 mg
- Children 1 to 3 years, 1.0 mg
  4 to 6 years, 1.1 mg
  7 to 10 years, 1.4 mg
- Males 11 to 14 years, 1.7 mg
  15 years and older, 2.0 mg
- Females 11 to 14 years, 1.4 mg
  15 to 18 years, 1.5 mg
  19 years and older, 1.6 mg
- Pregnant women, 2.2 mg
- Nursing women, 2.1 mg

Severe deficiencies of vitamin B$_6$ are rare, but mild deficiencies are extremely common. In a survey of 11,658 adults, 71% of men and 90% of women were found to have diets deficient in B$_6$.[1] Vitamin B$_6$ is the most commonly deficient water soluble vitamin in the elderly,[2] and children, too, don't get enough.[3]

Dietary deficiency can be worsened by use of hydralazine (for high blood pressure), penicillamine (used for rheumatoid arthritis and certain rare diseases), theophylline (an older drug for asthma), and the antituberculosis drug isoniazid (INH), all of which are thought to interfere with B$_6$ to some degree.[4-11] Good sources of B$_6$ include nutritional (torula) yeast, brewer's yeast, sunflower seeds, wheat germ, soybeans, walnuts, lentils, lima beans, buckwheat flour, bananas, and avocados.

Therapeutic Dosages

When used therapeutically, B$_6$ is commonly recommended at a daily dose of 10 to 300 mg daily, much higher than the basic nutritional requirement. However, it's probably not wise to take more than 50 mg daily, except on a physician's advice (see Safety Issues).

Since the B vitamins tend to work together, many nutritional experts recommend taking B$_6$ with other B vitamins, perhaps in the form of a B-complex supplement.

Therapeutic Uses

There is impressive evidence that an intake of vitamin B$_6$ somewhat above the Recommended Dietary Allowance levels (4.6 mg or more daily) can significantly reduce the risk of heart disease.[12]

A large double-blind study suggests that a higher dose (30 mg daily) of vitamin B$_6$ can reduce the nausea of morning sickness.[13]

Other common uses of B$_6$ are not very well established. For example, vitamin B$_6$ is widely recommended by conventional physicians as a treatment for carpal tunnel syndrome. However, there is little to no evidence that it actually works.[14] Similarly, although B_6 is frequently suggested as a treatment for PMS (premenstrual syndrome), there is some fairly good evidence that it doesn't work for this purpose.[15]

Some natural medicine authorities state that vitamin B_6 is a useful treatment for diabetic neuropathy. This idea is based on the fact that B_6 deficiency can cause neuropathy, and people with diabetes may be low in B_6. However, there is clinical evidence that B_6 supplements do not help diabetic neuropathy.[16,17,18]

Very weak evidence suggests that B6 may be helpful for depression,[19] allergy to monosodium glutamate (MSG, a highly allergenic food additive used to enhance flavor), asthma,[20,21] diabetes caused by pregnancy (gestational diabetes),[22] and kidney stones.[23,24,25] Finally, an interesting series of studies suggests (but certainly doesn't prove) that the combination of vitamin B_6 and magnesium can be helpful in autism.[26]

What Is the Scientific Evidence for Vitamin B₆?

Prevention of Atherosclerosis/Heart Disease

According to data gathered in the Nurses' Health Study, one of the largest long-term medical studies ever performed, vitamin B_6 supplements can significantly reduce a woman's risk of developing heart disease.[27] A total of 80,000 women with no history of heart disease were studied for possible links between vitamin B_6, folate, and the development of heart disease. The results showed that increased intake of B_6 could significantly reduce the risk of heart disease. Folate was also effective. (For more information, see the chapter on folate.)

Vitamin B_6 reduces blood levels of *homocysteine,* a chemical that has been linked to hardening of the arteries and heart disease. At first, it was assumed that the benefits of vitamin B_6 were all due to reducing homocysteine. However, a subsequent study found *no* association between high homocysteine levels and the risk of heart disease.[28] Instead, researchers found a connection between heart disease and low levels of vitamin B_6. People with the highest vitamin B_6 levels were 28% less likely to develop heart disease than those with the lowest B$_6$ levels. This study has led to the hypothesis that it is vitamin B$_6$ itself that reduces heart disease risk, and the reduction of homocysteine seen at the same time is simply incidental. However, the matter remains controversial.

Vitamin B$_6$ may help the heart in several ways. Preliminary studies suggest that it can reduce the tendency of platelets in the blood to form clots,[29] and also lower blood pressure to some extent.[30]

Morning Sickness (Nausea and Vomiting in Pregnancy)

Vitamin B$_6$ supplements have been used for years by conventional physicians as a treatment for morning sickness. In 1995, a large double-blind study validated this use.[31] A total of 342 pregnant women were given placebo or 30 mg of vitamin B$_6$ daily. Subjects then graded their symptoms by noting the severity of their nausea and recording the number of vomiting episodes. The women in the B$_6$ group experienced significantly less nausea than those in the placebo group, suggesting that regular use of B$_6$ can be helpful for morning sickness. However, vomiting episodes were not significantly reduced.

Premenstrual Syndrome (PMS)

More than a dozen double-blind studies investigated the effectiveness of vitamin B$_6$ for premenstrual syndrome (PMS). Many of these studies reported positive results, but a careful review of the literature found serious flaws in nearly all of them, so the results can't be taken as reliable.[32]

A recent properly designed double-blind trial of 120 women found *no* benefit.[33] In this study, three prescription antidepressants were compared against vitamin B$_6$ (pyridoxine, at 300 mg daily) and placebo. All study participants received 3 months of treatment and 3 months of placebo. Although the antidepressants were effective, vitamin B$_6$ proved to be no better than placebo.

Autism

According to four double-blind controlled trials, the combination of B$_6$ and magnesium may be helpful in autism.[34]

Sixty autistic children were treated with either B_6 alone, B_6 plus magnesium, or magnesium alone. Researchers found a modest benefit in behavior among the children taking both magnesium and B_6, but not in either of the other groups.

Asthma

A double-blind study of 76 children with asthma found significant benefit from vitamin B_6 after the second month of usage.[35] Children in the vitamin B_6 group were able to reduce their doses of asthma medication (bronchodilators and steroids). However, a recent double-blind study of 31 adults who used either inhaled or oral steroids did *not* show any benefit.[36] The dosages of B_6 used in these studies were quite high, in the range of 200 to 300 mg daily. Because of the risk of nerve injury, it is not advisable to take this much B_6 without medical supervision (see Safety Issues).

Safety Issues

Vitamin B_6 appears to be completely safe for adults at dosages up to 50 mg daily. However, at higher dosages (especially above 2 g daily) there is a very real risk of nerve damage. Nerve-related symptoms have even been reported at doses as low as 200 mg.[37] (This is a bit ironic, given that B_6 deficiency also causes nerve problems.) In some cases, very high doses of vitamin B_6 can cause or worsen acne symptoms.[38,39]

Maximum safe dosages for children, pregnant or nursing women, or those with severe liver or kidney disease have not been established.

⚠ Interactions You Should Know About

If you are taking

- **Isoniazid (INH)**, **penicillamine**, **hydralazine**, **oral contraceptives**, **phenelzine**, or **theophylline:** You may need extra vitamin B_6, but take only nutritional doses. Higher doses of B_6 might interfere with the action of the drug.
- **Levodopa** (for Parkinson's disease): Do not take more than 5 mg of vitamin B_6 daily except on medical advice.[40]

VITAMIN B$_{12}$

Supplement Forms/Alternate Names
Cobalamin, Cyanocobalamin, Hydrocobalamin, Methylcobalamin
Principal Proposed Uses
Pernicious Anemia, Correcting Absorption Problems Caused by
Medications
Other Proposed Uses
Male Infertility, Asthma, AIDS, Diabetic Neuropathy, Multiple Sclerosis,
Tinnitus, Alzheimer's Disease, Depression, Osteoporosis, Periodontal
Disease

Vitamin B$_{12}$, an essential nutrient, is also known as cobalamin. The "cobal" in the name refers to the metal cobalt contained in B$_{12}$. Vitamin B$_{12}$ is required for the normal activity
of nerve cells, and works with folate and vitamin B$_6$ to lower
blood levels of *homocysteine,* a chemical in the blood that is
thought to contribute to heart disease. (For more information about homocysteine and heart disease, see the chapters
on folate and vitamin B$_6$.) B$_{12}$ also plays a role in the body's
manufacture of S-adenosylmethionine, or SAMe (see the
chapter on SAMe).

Anemia is usually the first sign of B$_{12}$ deficiency. Earlier
in this century, doctors coined the name "pernicious anemia"
for a stubborn anemia that didn't improve even when the patient was given iron supplements. Today we know that pernicious anemia is usually caused by a condition in which the
stomach fails to excrete a special substance called intrinsic
factor. The body needs the intrinsic factor for efficient absorption of vitamin B$_{12}$. In 1948, vitamin B$_{12}$ was identified as
the cure for pernicious anemia.

More recent evidence suggests that B$_{12}$ supplements may
improve sperm count and mobility, possibly enhancing fertility. Vitamin B$_{12}$ has also been proposed as a treatment for numerous other conditions, but as yet there is no definitive
evidence that it is effective.

Requirements/Sources

Extraordinarily small amounts of vitamin B$_{12}$ suffice for daily nutritional needs. The U.S. Recommended Dietary Allowance is as follows

- Infants under 6 months, 0.3 mcg
    6 to 12 months, 0.5 mcg
- Children 1 to 3 years, 0.7 mcg
    4 to 6 years, 1.0 mcg
    7 to 10 years, 1.4 mcg
- Males and females 11 years and older, 2.0 mcg
- Pregnant women, 2.2 mcg
- Nursing women, 2.6 mcg

Vitamin B$_{12}$ deficiency is rare in the young, but it's not unusual in older people: Probably 10 to 20% of the elderly are deficient in B$_{12}$.[1-4] This may be because older people have lower levels of stomach acid. The vitamin B$_{12}$ in our food comes attached to proteins and must be released by acid in the stomach in order to be absorbed. When stomach acid levels are low, we don't absorb as much vitamin B$_{12}$ from our food. Fortunately, vitamin B$_{12}$ supplements don't need acid for absorption. For this reason, people who take medications that greatly reduce stomach acid, such as Prilosec (omeprazole) or Zantac (ranitidine), should probably also take B$_{12}$ supplements.[5-10]

Stomach surgery and other conditions affecting the digestive tract can also lead to B$_{12}$ deficiency. Vitamin B$_{12}$ absorption is also impaired by colchicine (for gout), metformin and phenformin (for diabetes), and bile acid sequestrants such as colestipol and cholestyramine (for high cholesterol).[11-15]

Slow-release potassium supplements can also impair B$_{12}$ absorption.[16]

Severe B$_{12}$ deficiency can cause anemia and, potentially, nerve damage. The latter may become permanent if the deficiency is not corrected in time. Anemia usually develops first, leading to treatment before permanent nerve damage develops. However, folate supplements can get in the way of this "early warning system." This is why people are cautioned against taking high doses of folate without medical supervision. When taken at a dosage higher than 400 mcg daily, folate can prevent anemia caused by B_{12} deficiency, thereby allowing permanent nerve damage to develop without any warning. Therefore, you should not take folate at high dosages without first getting a blood test to evaluate your B_{12} levels.

Vitamin B_{12} is found in most animal foods. Beef, liver, clams, and lamb provide a whopping 80 to 100 mcg of B_{12} per 3.5-ounce serving, at least 40 times the dietary requirement. Sardines, chicken liver, beef kidney, and calf liver are also good sources, providing between 25 and 60 mcg per serving. Trout, salmon, tuna, eggs, whey, and many cheeses provide at least the recommended daily intake. Nondairy, or total, vegetarians can eventually become B_{12}-deficient, unless they take B_{12} supplements or eat B_{12}-enriched yeast.

Vitamin B_{12} is available in three forms: cyanocobalamin, hydrocobalamin, and methylcobalamin. The first is the most widely available and least expensive, but some experts think that the other two forms are preferable.

Therapeutic Dosages

For correcting absorption problems caused by medications, taking vitamin B_{12} at the level of dietary requirements should suffice.

For other purposes, enormously higher daily doses—ranging from 100 to 2,000 mcg—are sometimes recommended.

Because the B vitamins tend to work together, many nutritional experts recommend taking B_{12} with other B vitamins in the form of a B-complex supplement.

Therapeutic Uses

It appears that individuals who take medications that dramatically lower stomach acid would profit by taking B_{12} supplements.[17–22]

For pernicious anemia, B_{12} injections are traditionally used but research has shown that oral B_{12} works just as well, provided you take enough of it (between 300 and 1,000 mcg daily).[23–26]

Preliminary evidence suggests that B_{12} supplements may improve sperm activity and sperm count and perhaps treat male infertility.[27,28]

Vitamin B_{12} is widely recommended as a treatment for asthma,[29] but there is little real evidence that it is effective. On the basis of weak and sometimes contradictory evidence, vitamin B_{12} has been suggested for AIDS,[30,31] diabetic neuropathy,[32,33] multiple sclerosis (MS),[34,35] and tinnitus.[36]

Although vitamin B_{12} has been proposed as a treatment for Alzheimer's disease, this recommendation is based solely on the results of one small, poorly designed study.[37] More recent and better-designed studies found little to no benefit.[38,39]

Vitamin B_{12} is also sometimes recommended for numerous other problems, including depression, osteoporosis, and periodontal disease, but there is little to no evidence as yet that it really works.

What Is the Scientific Evidence for Vitamin B_{12}?

Male Infertility

Vitamin B_{12} deficiencies in men can lead to reduced sperm counts and lowered sperm mobility. For this reason, B_{12} supplements have been tried for improving fertility in men with abnormal sperm production. In one double-blind study of 375 infertile men, supplementation with vitamin B_{12} produced no benefits on average in the group as a whole.[40] However, in a particular subgroup of men with sufficiently low sperm count and sperm motility, B_{12} appeared to be helpful. Such "dredging" of the data is suspect from a scientific point of view, however, and this study cannot be taken as proof of effectiveness.

Safety Issues

Vitamin B_{12} appears to be extremely safe. However, in some cases very high doses of vitamin B_{12} can cause or worsen acne symptoms.[41,42]

⚠ Interactions You Should Know About

If you are taking

- Medications that reduce stomach acid such as **H_2 blockers** (e.g., Zantac [ranitidine]) and **proton pump inhibitors** (e.g., Prilosec [omeprazole]), **colchicine**, **Glucophage (metformin)**, **phenformin**, **oral contraceptives**, **nitrous oxide**, **bile acid sequestrants** (e.g., Questran [cholestyramine] or Colestid [colestipol]), or **clofibrate:** You may need extra B_{12}.
- **Potassium:** You may need extra B_{12}.
- High doses of **vitamin C:** Blood tests for vitamin B_{12} may not be reliable.

VITAMIN C

Supplement Forms/Alternate Names
Ascorbate, Ascorbic Acid

Principal Proposed Uses
Colds, Cataracts, Macular Degeneration

Other Proposed Uses
Preeclampsia Prevention, Asthma, Hypertension, Bedsores, Low Sperm Count, Sunburn Prevention, Alzheimer's Disease, Diabetes, Hepatitis, Herpes, Insomnia, Parkinson's Disease, Periodontal Disease, Rheumatoid Arthritis, Bladder Infection, Menopausal Symptoms, Migraine Headaches, Nausea, Ulcers, Allergies, Cancer Prevention, Cancer Treatment, Heart Disease Prevention, Osteoarthritis, General Antioxidant

Although most animals can make vitamin C from scratch, humans have lost the ability. We must get it from food, chiefly fresh fruits and vegetables. One of this vitamin's main functions is helping the body manufacture collagen, a key protein in our connective tissues, cartilage, and tendons.

From ancient times through the early nineteenth century, sailors and others deprived of fresh fruits and vegetables developed a disease called *scurvy*. Scurvy involves so-called scorbutic symptoms, which include nonhealing wounds, bleeding gums, bruising, and overall weakness. Now we know that scurvy is nothing more than vitamin C deficiency.

Scurvy was successfully treated with citrus fruit during the mid-1700s. In 1928, when Albert Szent-Gyorgyi isolated the active ingredient, he called it the "anti-scorbutic principle," or ascorbic acid. This, of course, is vitamin C.

Vitamin C is a powerful antioxidant that protects against damaging natural substances called free radicals. It works in water, both inside and outside of cells. Vitamin C complements another antioxidant vitamin, vitamin E, which works in lipid (fatty) parts of the body.

Vitamin C is the single most popular vitamin supplement in the United States, and perhaps the most controversial as well. In the 1960s, two-time Nobel Prize winner Dr. Linus Pauling claimed that vitamin C could effectively treat both cancer and the common cold. Research has been mixed on both counts, but that hasn't dampened enthusiasm for this essential nutrient. The vitamin C movement has led to hundreds of clinical studies testing the vitamin on dozens of illnesses.

Requirements/Sources

Vitamin C is an essential nutrient that must be obtained from food or supplements—the body cannot manufacture it. The U.S. Recommended Dietary Allowance is as follows

- Infants under 6 months, 30 mg
  6 to 12 months, 35 mg
- Children 1 to 3 years, 40 mg
  4 to 10 years, 45 mg
  11 to 14 years, 50 mg
- Adults (and teenagers 15 years and older), 60 mg
- Pregnant women, 70 mg
- Nursing women, 90 to 95 mg

Scurvy, the classic vitamin C deficiency disease, is now a rarity in the developed world, although a more subtle deficiency of vitamin C is fairly common, especially among hospital patients.[1-4] Also, aspirin and possibly other anti-inflammatory drugs can lower body levels of vitamin C.[5,6,7]

Most of us think of orange juice as the quintessential source of vitamin C, but many vegetables are actually even richer sources. Red chili peppers, sweet peppers, kale, parsley, collard, and turnip greens are excellent sources, as are broccoli, brussels sprouts, watercress, cauliflower, cabbage, and strawberries. (Oranges and other citrus fruits are good sources, too.)

One great advantage of getting vitamin C from foods rather than from supplements is that you will get many other healthy nutrients at the same time, such as bioflavonoids and carotenes. However, vitamin C in food is partially destroyed by cooking and exposure to air, so for maximum nutritional benefit you might want to try freshly made salads rather than dishes that require a lot of cooking.

Vitamin C supplements are available in two forms: ascorbic acid and ascorbate. The latter is less intensely sour.

Therapeutic Dosages

Ever since Linus Pauling, proponents have recommended taking vitamin C in enormous doses, as high as 20 to 30 g daily. However, some evidence suggests that there might not be any reason to take more than 200 mg of vitamin C daily (10 to 100 times less than the amount recommended by vitamin C proponents).[8] The reason is that if you consume more than 200 mg daily (researchers have tested up to 2,500 mg) your kidneys begin to excrete the excess at a steadily increasing rate, matching the increased dose. Your digestive tract also stops absorbing it well. The net effect is that no matter how much you take, your blood levels of vitamin C don't increase.

However, there are some flaws in this research. It is possible that vitamin C levels might rise in other tissues even if they remain constant in the blood. Furthermore, this study did not take into account the effects of taking vitamin C several times daily.

Many nutritional experts recommend a total of 500 mg of vitamin C daily. This dose is almost undoubtedly safe. Others recommend that you take as much vitamin C as you can, up to 30,000 mg daily, cutting back only when you start to develop stomach cramps and diarrhea. This recommendation is not so much based on any evidence that such huge doses of vitamin C are good for you, but primarily on a semireligious enthusiasm.

Therapeutic Uses

According to numerous double-blind studies, vitamin C supplements can reduce symptoms of colds and shorten the length of the illness.[9,10]

A sizable double-blind study suggests that the use of vitamin C and vitamin E supplements can reduce the risk of developing preeclampsia, a complication of pregnancy.[11]

Observational studies (studies in which researchers observe the participants to try to identify lifestyle factors associated with better health) tell us that people who regularly use vitamin C supplements are less likely to develop either of two eye problems, cataracts and macular degeneration.[12–17]

Many studies have tried to evaluate whether vitamin C supplements can help asthma, and although the results have been mixed, on balance the evidence suggests that vitamin C may be slightly helpful.[18] The same may be said of using vitamin C to treat hypertension.[19,20]

Small double-blind studies suggest that vitamin C may be able to speed recovery from bedsores.[21] Vitamin C may improve sperm count and function;[22] however, a recent double-blind study of 31 individuals found no benefit.[23] When combined with vitamin E, vitamin C may help prevent sunburn.[24,25] In addition, vitamin C supplements have been recommended for Alzheimer's disease, bladder infections, diabetes, hepatitis, herpes, insomnia, menopausal symptoms, migraine headaches, nausea, Parkinson's disease, periodontal disease, rheumatoid arthritis, and ulcers, but there is no solid scientific basis for any of these uses.

Vitamin C is often suggested as a treatment for allergies, but the research results are very preliminary and somewhat contradictory.[26,27,28]

Vitamin C in the diet appears to reduce the risk of cancer and heart disease and slow the progression of osteoarthritis.[29,30] However, there is little evidence that vitamin C *supplements* provide the same benefits. As noted earlier, foods containing vitamin C also contain many other healthful ingredients (such as bioflavonoids and carotenes), so it's not clear that pills containing vitamin C alone work just as well.

Vitamin C has been proposed as a treatment for cancer, but this claim is very controversial, and there is as yet no scientifically meaningful evidence that it works.[31–34]

According to a double-blind placebo-controlled study of 141 women with cervical dysplasia (early cervical cancer), vitamin C, taken at a dosage of 500 mg daily, does not help to reverse the dysplasia.[35]

Heated disagreement exists regarding whether it is safe or appropriate to combine vitamin C with standard chemotherapy drugs.[36,37] The reasoning behind this concern is that many chemotherapy drugs work in part by creating free radicals that destroy cancer cells. Antioxidants like vitamin C might interfere with this beneficial effect. Indeed, some cancer cells appear to accumulate vitamin C to protect themselves from injury! On the other hand, some evidence suggests that vitamin C may help reduce the side effects of certain chemotherapy drugs without decreasing their effectiveness.[38,39] Nonetheless, in view of the high stakes involved, we strongly recommend that you do not take any supplements while undergoing cancer chemotherapy except on the advice of a physician.

What Is the Scientific Evidence for Vitamin C?

Colds

As the most famous of all natural treatments for colds, vitamin C has been subjected to irresponsible hype from both proponents and opponents. Enthusiasts claim that if you take vitamin C daily, you will never get sick, while enemies of the treatment insist that vitamin C has no benefit at all.

However, a cool-headed evaluation of the research indicates something in between. Numerous studies have found that vitamin C supplements taken at a dose of 1,000 mg daily or more can significantly reduce symptoms of colds and help you get over a cold faster.[40,41,42] Benefits appear to be greater for children than for adults, and the exact amount of the benefit varies widely between studies.

In most of these studies, participants took vitamin C supplements on a daily basis throughout the period of the study.[43] However, a few studies evaluated the benefits of taking vitamin C only right at the onset of cold symptoms. This method, which is perhaps the most popular way of using vitamin C for colds, appears to be just as effective.

There is no real evidence that vitamin C supplements can prevent colds in general. However, there are two exceptions to this. One is the "post-marathon sniffle." Heavy endurance exercise temporarily weakens the immune system, leading to a high incidence of infection following marathons and triathlons. There is some evidence that vitamin C can prevent such colds.[44,45]

The other situation in which vitamin C may help prevent colds is when you are actually *deficient* in the vitamin. There is some evidence that making sure to get your dietary allowance might help keep you healthier.[46]

Cataracts

Regular use of vitamin C may reduce the risk of cataracts, probably by fighting free radicals that damage the lens of the eye. In an observational study of 50,800 nurses followed for 8 years, it was found that people who used vitamin C supplements for more than 10 years had a 45% lower rate of cataract development.[47] Interestingly, diets high in vitamin C were not found to be protective—only supplemental vitamin C made a difference. This is the opposite of what has been found with vitamin C in the prevention of other diseases, such as cancer (see the section titled Cancer Prevention).

A more recent study of 247 women suggests that vitamin C supplements taken for more than 10 years reduce the incidence of cataracts by 77%.[48] In this study, no benefit was found for shorter-term vitamin C supplementation.

It has been suggested that vitamin C may be particularly useful against cataracts in people with diabetes, because of its influence on *sorbitol,* a sugar-like substance that tends to accumulate in the cells of diabetics. Excess sorbitol is believed to play a role in the development of diabetes-related cataracts, and vitamin C appears to help reduce sorbitol buildup.[49]

Macular Degeneration

After cataracts, injury to the macula (the most important part of the retina) is the second most common cause of vision loss in people 65 and older.

Observational studies involving a total of over 4,000 people suggest that regular use of vitamin C supplements may help prevent macular degeneration.[50,51] Vitamin C is thought to work by protecting the retina against damaging free radicals.

According to one study, a combination of many antioxidants including vitamin C might be able to halt macular degeneration that has already begun. In this 18-month, double-blind trial, a daily supplement containing 750 mg of vitamin C, 200 IU of vitamin E, 50 mcg of selenium, and 20,000 IU of beta-carotene (along with other ingredients) actually stopped progression of macular degeneration.[52]

Warning: If you have macular degeneration, do not self-treat it without first seeing a physician. One particular type of macular degeneration must be treated with laser surgery.

Preeclampsia Prevention

Preeclampsia is a dangerous complication of pregnancy that involves high blood pressure, swelling of the whole body, and improper kidney function. A double-blind placebo-controlled study of 283 women at increased risk for preeclampsia found that supplementation with vitamin C (1,000 mg daily) and vitamin E (400 IU daily) significantly reduced the chances for developing this disease.[53]

While this research is promising, larger studies are necessary to confirm whether vitamins C and E will actually work. The authors of this study point out that similarly sized studies found benefits with other treatments, such as aspirin, that later proved to be ineffective when large-scale studies were performed. Furthermore, keep in mind that we don't know whether such high dosages of these vitamins are absolutely safe for pregnant women.

Cancer Prevention

While there is some evidence that dietary vitamin C from fruits and vegetables can reduce the risk of cancer, we don't know if vitamin C *supplements* are particularly helpful. This is a crucial distinction. When you get vitamin C from fruits and vegetables, you also receive myriad other substances such as bioflavonoids and carotenes that may provide health benefits. The studies involving vitamin C supplements and cancer prevention have not shown stellar results.

One study found that vitamin C supplementation at 500 mg or more daily was connected to a lower incidence of bladder cancer.[54] However, another study found *no* benefit.[55]

Supplemental vitamin C at 1 g daily failed to prevent new colon cancers after one had developed.[56] In another large observational study, 500 mg or more of vitamin C daily over a period of 6 years provided no significant protection against breast cancer.[57] Another study found similar results.[58]

Cancer Treatment

Cancer treatment is one of the more controversial proposed uses of vitamin C. An early study tested vitamin C in 1,100 terminally ill cancer patients. One hundred patients received 10 g daily of vitamin C, while 1,000 other patients (the control group) received no treatment. Those taking the vitamin survived more than 4 times longer on average (210 days) than those in the control group (50 days).[59] A large (1,826 subjects) follow-up study by the same researchers found a nearly doubled survival rate (343 days versus 180 days) in vitamin C–treated patients whose cancers were deemed "incurable," as compared to untreated controls.[60] However, these studies were poorly designed, and other generally better constructed studies have found no benefit of vitamin C in cancer.[61,62] At the present time, vitamin C cannot be regarded as a proven treatment for cancer.

Heart Disease Prevention

As with cancer prevention, there is some evidence that eating vitamin C–rich foods can reduce your risk of heart disease. However, the evidence that vitamin C supplements taken by themselves are helpful for atherosclerosis is weak.[63,64,65] A combination of supplemental vitamins C and E may offer some heart-protective benefits, although the evidence for this comes only from observational studies.[66]

Hypertension (High Blood Pressure)

According to a 30-day, double-blind study of 39 individuals taking medications for hypertension, treatment with 500 mg of vitamin C daily can reduce blood pressure by about 10%.[67] However, another double-blind study, which involved 48 individuals given the same amount of vitamin C, found no benefit.[68] Other studies on the subject have been of generally poor quality.[69,70,71]

Safety Issues

Vitamin C is indisputably safe at dosages up to 500 mg daily, and is probably not dangerous at much higher doses. Reports that vitamin C can cause DNA damage were based on an exaggerated interpretation of a fairly theoretical finding.[72]

If you take more than 1,000 to 2,000 mg daily, you may develop diarrhea. This side effect may go away with continued use of vitamin C, but you may have to cut down your dosage for a while, and then gradually build up again. At a high enough dosage, however, the diarrhea can continue indefinitely as long as you keep taking the vitamin C. Staying below this amount is called "taking vitamin C to bowel tolerance." As mentioned earlier though, there may not be much point to taking more than 200 to 500 mg of vitamin C daily.

High-dose vitamin C can cause copper deficiency and excessive iron absorption.

Additionally, there is reason for concern that long-term vitamin C treatment can cause kidney stones,[73] However, in large-scale studies the people who took the most vitamin C (over 1,500 mg daily) actually had a *lower* risk of kidney stones than those taking the least amounts.[74,75,76] Nonetheless, people with a history of kidney stones and those with kidney failure who have a defect in vitamin C or oxalate metabolism should probably restrict vitamin C intake to approximately 100 mg daily.[77]

You should also avoid high-dose vitamin C if you have glucose-6-phosphate dehydrogenase deficiency, iron overload, kidney failure, or a history of intestinal surgery. Vitamin C may also reduce the blood-thinning effects of Coumadin (warfarin) and heparin.[78,79]

The maximum safe dosages of vitamin C for young children, pregnant or nursing women, or those with severe liver or kidney disease have not been determined.

⚠ Interactions You Should Know About

If you are taking

- **Aspirin** or other **anti-inflammatory drugs**, **oral contraceptives**, or e**strogen-replacement therapy:** You may need more vitamin C.
- **Coumadin (warfarin)** or **heparin:** High-dose vitamin C might reduce their effectiveness.
- **Iron supplements:** High-dose vitamin C can cause you to absorb too much iron. This is especially a problem for people with diseases that cause them to store too much iron.
- High doses of **vitamin C:** Your ability to absorb copper may be impaired, and tests for vitamin B_{12} levels may not be accurate.

VITAMIN D

Supplement Forms/Alternate Names
Cholecalciferol (Vitamin D$_3$), Ergocalciferol (Vitamin D$_2$)

Principal Proposed Uses
Preventing and Treating Osteoporosis

Other Proposed Uses
Cancer Prevention, Psoriasis

Vitamin D is both a vitamin and a hormone. It's a vitamin because your body cannot absorb calcium without it; it's a hormone because your body manufactures it in response to your skin's exposure to sunlight.

There are two major forms of vitamin D, and both have the word *calciferol* in their names. In Latin, *calciferol* means "calcium carrier." Vitamin D$_3$ (cholecalciferol) is made by the body and is found in some foods. Vitamin D$_2$ (ergocalciferol) is the form most often added to milk and other foods, and the form you're most likely to use as a supplement.

Strong evidence tells us that the combination of vitamin D and calcium supplements can be quite helpful for preventing and treating osteoporosis.

Requirements/Sources

As with vitamin A and vitamin E, dosages of vitamin D are often expressed in terms of international units (IU) rather than milligrams. The adequate intake (AI) for vitamin D is as follows

- Infants under 6 months, 200 IU (5 mcg) daily
- Males and females 6 months to 50 years, 200 IU (5 mcg)
      51 to 70 years, 400 IU (10 mcg)
      71 years and older, 600 IU (15 mcg)
- Pregnant women, 200 IU (5 mcg)
- Nursing women, 200 IU (5 mcg)

One researcher has given a strong argument that these recommendations are too low and should be increased considerably, perhaps by as much as a factor of 10.[1] However, this idea has not been universally accepted, and some authorities feel that vitamin D toxicity is a real risk.[2]

There is very little vitamin D found naturally in the foods we eat (the best sources are coldwater fish). In many countries, vitamin D is added to milk and other foods like breakfast cereals and margarine, contributing to our daily intake.

By far the best source of vitamin D is sunlight. However, in view of current recommendations stressing sunblock and sun avoidance, we can't advise you to get your vitamin D this way. It is interesting to note that severe vitamin D deficiency was common in England in the 1800s due to coal smoke obscuring the sun. Cod liver oil, which is high in vitamin D, became popular as a children's supplement to help prevent rickets. (Rickets is a disease in which developing bones soften and curve because they aren't receiving enough calcium.) It is possible that recent emphasis on avoiding the sun will have some negative consequences.

Vitamin D deficiency is known to occur in the elderly as well as in people who live in northern latitudes and don't drink vitamin D–enriched milk.[3,4] Women with significant osteoporosis are also often vitamin D deficient.[5] Additionally, phenytoin, primidone, and phenobarbital (for seizures); corticosteroids; cimetidine (for ulcers); and the antituberculosis drug isoniazid (INH) may interfere with vitamin D absorption or activity.[6–14]

Therapeutic Dosages

For therapeutic purposes, vitamin D is taken at the nutritional doses described in Requirements/Sources (and sometimes at even higher amounts). If you wish to exceed nutritional levels of vitamin D intake, physician supervision is recommended (see Safety Issues).

Therapeutic Uses

Without question, if you are concerned about osteoporosis, you should take calcium and vitamin D. The combination definitely helps prevent bone loss.[15,16] This is true even if you are taking estrogen or any other treatment for osteoporosis; after all, you can't build bone without calcium, and you can't properly absorb and utilize calcium without adequate intake of vitamin D. Other uses of vitamin D are less well documented. Some evidence suggests that vitamin D may help prevent cancer of the breast, colon, pancreas, and prostate, but the research on this question has yielded mixed results.[17–23]

Vitamin D is sometimes mentioned as a treatment for psoriasis. However, this recommendation is based on Danish studies using calcipotriol, a variation of vitamin D_3 that is used externally (applied to the skin).[24] Calcipotriol does *not* affect your body's absorption of calcium, so it is a very different substance from the vitamin D you can purchase at a store.

What Is the Scientific Evidence for Vitamin D?

Osteoporosis

Women with severe osteoporosis have low levels of vitamin D.[25] Supplementing with vitamin D alone may not be helpful,[26] but the combination of calcium and vitamin D can slow down or even reverse osteoporosis.

One double-blind study followed 249 women in Boston for 1 year; the location of this study is important because your body can't produce significant amounts of vitamin D from sunlight during the winter in Boston.[27] These were postmenopausal women with an average age of 61, none of whom were taking estrogen or other medications for bone loss. Half of the women received a calcium citrate malate supplement (400 mg daily) plus a vitamin D supplement (400 IU daily), while the other half received placebo. The women in this study who were taking the vitamin D and calcium experienced a net increase in spinal bone mass (0.85%), while the placebo group showed no net change—a significant difference.

Another double-blind placebo-controlled study enrolling 3,270 women (nearly all of whom had never been on estrogen-replacement therapy) found that higher dosages of vitamin D produced even better results. For a period of 1½ years, participants received either placebo or 1,200 mg of calcium and 800 IU of vitamin D. At the end of the study period, the researchers found that the bone density in the hips of the women who had taken calcium and vitamin D had increased by 2.7%, while the hip bone density of the women who had taken placebo *decreased* by 4.6%. The calcium/vitamin D group also had 43% fewer hip fractures. A reduced fracture rate was also seen in another large, double-blind placebo-controlled study.[28]

There is also some good evidence that the use of calcium combined with vitamin D can help protect against the bone loss caused by corticosteroid drugs (such as prednisone). In a 2-year, double-blind placebo-controlled study of 130 individuals, supplementation with 1,000 mg of calcium and 500 IU of vitamin D daily actually reversed steroid-induced bone loss, causing a net bone gain.[29]

Safety Issues

When taken at recommended dosages, vitamin D appears to be safe. However, when used at considerable excess, vitamin D can build up in the body and cause toxic symptoms. According to current recommendations, the maximum safe dosage of vitamin D, in the absence of sunlight or other sources, is 2,000 IU daily. However, the actual dosage at which intake becomes toxic is a matter of dispute.[30,31]

People with sarcoidosis or hyperparathyroidism should never take vitamin D without first consulting a physician.

⚠ Interactions You Should Know About

If you are taking

- **Antiseizure drugs (phenobarbital, primidone, valproic acid, or phenytoin), corticosteroids, heparin, isoniazid (INH), or rifampin:** You may need extra vitamin D.

- **Thiazide diuretics:** Do not take calcium and vitamin D supplements unless under a doctor's supervision.

VITAMIN E

Supplement Forms/Alternate Names

Alpha Tocopherol, D-Alpha-Tocopherol, D-Beta-Tocopherol, D-Delta-Tocopherol, D-Gamma-Tocopherol, D-Tocopherol, DL-Alpha-Tocopherol, DL-Tocopherol, Mixed Tocopherols, Tocopheryl Acetate, Tocopheryl Succinate

Principal Proposed Uses

Cancer Prevention

Other Proposed Uses

Heart Disease Prevention, Preeclampsia Prevention, Tardive Dyskinesia, Diabetes, Sunburn Prevention, Impaired Immunity, Alzheimer's Disease, Rheumatoid Arthritis, Male Infertility, Cataracts, Macular Degeneration, Osteoarthritis, PMS, Bodybuilding Exercise, Asthma, Acne, Gout, Psoriasis, Angina, Reduction of Amiodarone Side Effects

---

Vitamin E is an antioxidant that fights damaging natural substances known as free radicals. It works in lipids (fats and oils), which makes it complementary to vitamin C, which fights free radicals dissolved in water.

There is evidence that vitamin E can prevent certain forms of cancer. Vitamin E has also shown considerable promise for preventing preeclampsia (a complication of pregnancy), treating tardive dyskinesia (a side effect of antipsychotic drugs), improving immunity, slowing the progression of Alzheimer's disease, and improving male fertility. However, contrary to earlier indications, vitamin E does not appear to prevent heart disease.

Requirements/Sources

The U.S. Recommended Dietary Allowance for vitamin E is measured not in milligrams but in international units (IU) and is as follows

- Infants under 6 months, 3 IU
  6 months to 1 year, 4 IU

- Children 1 to 3 years, 6 IU
    4 to 6 years, 7 IU
    7 to 10 years, 7 IU
- Males 11 years and older, 10 IU
- Females 11 years and older, 8 IU
- Pregnant women, 10 IU
- Nursing women, 11 to 12 IU

In developed countries, dietary deficiency of vitamin E is relatively common.[1,2,3] Vitamin E is actually a family of compounds called *tocopherols*. While there are many tocopherols, the most common form used in supplements is a synthetic form called *dl-alpha tocopherol*. However, there is some evidence that natural forms of vitamin E are more effective.[4,5,6] Natural-source vitamin E contains beta-, delta-, and gamma-tocopherols, as well as other compounds in the tocopherol family (such as tocotrienols). Natural vitamin E also differs from the synthetic kind in another way as well. Natural vitamin E comes in a form called a d-isomer (the "d" stands for *dextro*, or right-handed). Synthetic vitamin E contains a mixture of d- and l-isomers ("l" is for *levo*, or left-handed).

It has been suggested that the best vitamin E supplement would be a natural mixture of tocopherols including alpha, delta, and gamma ("mixed tocopherols"), all of which should be in the "d" form. However, all the scientific evidence we have for the effectiveness of vitamin E supplements comes from studies using synthetic dl-alpha-tocopherol, so at this point we have no direct confirmation that natural vitamin E is better.

The best food sources of vitamin E are polyunsaturated vegetable oils, seeds, nuts, and whole grains. To get a therapeutic dosage, though, you need to take a supplement.

Therapeutic Dosages

The optimal therapeutic dosage of vitamin E has not been established. Most studies have used between 50 and 800 IU daily, and some have used even higher doses.

If you wish to purchase natural vitamin E, look for a label that says "mixed tocopherols." However, some manufacturers use this term to mean the synthetic dl-alpha tocopherol, so you need to read the contents closely. Natural tocopherols come as d-alpha-, d-gamma-, d-delta-, and d-beta-tocopherol.

Therapeutic Uses

Vitamin E appears to help prevent various forms of cancer, especially prostate[7] and colon[8] cancer.

Vitamin E might be slightly helpful for angina.[9] However, contrary to earlier indications, it does not seem to help prevent heart disease.[10]

Vitamin E appears to reduce symptoms of tardive dyskinesia, an unpleasant movement disorder that can develop after years of taking antipsychotic drugs.[11–15]

When combined with vitamin C, vitamin E appears to help prevent sunburn.[16,17]

Intriguing evidence suggests that vitamin E may also prevent preeclampsia,[18] improve immunity,[19] slow the progression of Alzheimer's disease,[20] reduce pain in rheumatoid arthritis,[21] improve symptoms of diabetic neuropathy,[22,23] and help protect people with diabetes from developing damage to their eyes and kidneys.[24] Vitamin E may also be helpful in treating male infertility,[25] although a recent double-blind study of 31 individuals found no benefit.[26] Weaker evidence suggests that vitamin E can prevent cataracts,[27–30] improve blood sugar control in people with type 2 diabetes,[31,32,33] help prevent or treat macular degeneration, slow the progression of osteoarthritis,[34] and reduce symptoms of PMS.[35,36]

There is also some evidence that vitamin E may be useful during weight training.[37] Heavy exercise produces free radicals that can disrupt the muscles and cause pain. Vitamin E appears to exert a protective effect in this regard.

Additionally, vitamin E might help reduce the lung-related side effects caused by the drug amiodarone (used to prevent abnormal heart rhythms).[38]

Vitamin E does *not* appear to be helpful for cyclic breast pain, sometimes called fibrocystic breast disease, cyclic mastitis, or cyclic mastalgia.[39] In addition, despite some claims to the contrary, supplemental vitamin E does not seem to be helpful for treating Parkinson's disease.[40,41] It might, however, be useful for *preventing* Parkinson's disease.[42]

Vitamin E and other antioxidants are frequently recommended for asthma, on the grounds that they may protect inflamed lung tissue, but there is no scientific evidence that they work. Similarly, although vitamin E has been suggested as a treatment for acne, gout, and psoriasis, there is no real supporting evidence for any of these uses.

Although vitamin E is often recommended for menopausal hot flashes, there is no real evidence that it is effective. One 9-week, double-blind placebo-controlled trial followed 104 women with hot flashes associated with breast cancer treatment, but it found marginal benefits at best.[43]

What Is the Scientific Evidence for Vitamin E?

Cancer Prevention

Vitamin E appears to offer dramatic benefits for preventing prostate and colon cancer. In an intervention trial that involved 29,133 smokers, those who were given about 50 IU of vitamin E daily for 5 to 8 years showed a 32% lower incidence of prostate cancer, a 41% drop in prostate cancer deaths, and a 16% decrease in the incidence of colon cancer.[44]

Surprisingly, these benefits were seen fairly soon after the start of supplementation, even though prostate cancer is very slow growing. A cancer that shows up today had its start many years ago. The fact that vitamin E almost immediately lowered the incidence of prostate cancer suggests that it somehow blocks the step at which a hidden prostate cancer makes the leap into becoming detectable.

The dosage of vitamin E used in this study was lower than what is usually recommended. It is quite reasonable to assume that a higher dosage would be more effective, but this has not been proven.

Vitamin E may be even more effective in people who do not smoke. Researchers at the Fred Hutchinson Cancer Research Center in Seattle found that regular use of supplemental vitamin E (200 IU or more daily) cut colon cancer risk by 57%.[45] Another observational study found a 29 to 59% reduction, based on the length of time vitamin E was used.[46]

Heart Disease

The latest research findings appear to have turned the tables on our once high hopes for vitamin E. Now it looks increasingly unlikely that this antioxidant vitamin is a "magic bullet" that by itself can put a dent in heart disease.

The Heart Outcomes Prevention Evaluation (HOPE) trial found that natural vitamin E (d-alpha tocopherol) at a dose of 400 IU daily did not reduce the number of heart attacks, strokes, or deaths from heart disease any more than a placebo.[47] The details of this well-designed double-blind trial were published in the January 20, 2000 issue of *The New England Journal of Medicine*. The trial, lasting an average of 4.5 years, followed over 9,000 men and women who had existing heart disease or were at high risk for it.

We already knew that vitamin E supplements (50 IU) didn't work for heart disease in smokers,[48,49,50] but that could be readily explained away: Perhaps vitamin E, especially in that relatively small dose, could not overcome the damaging effects of smoking.

The Cambridge Heart Antioxidant Study (CHAOS) trial,[51] published in 1996, is what really had gotten our hopes up. In that trial, people with existing heart disease who took natural vitamin E (400 IU or 800 IU daily) had substantially fewer nonfatal heart attacks compared to the placebo group after about 1.5 years. Even so, and this may resonate with the latest findings, heart-related deaths were not reduced in the vitamin E group. Furthermore, it has been suggested that possible flaws in the design of this trial might make its findings questionable.

Large observational studies in both men and women found substantial benefits for vitamin E (100 IU).[52,53,54] One observational study of 11,178 people aged 67 to 105 years found good results from combining vitamins E and C.[55] Those who were taking vitamin E supplements at the beginning of the study had a 34% lower risk of death from heart disease than those who were not. Vitamin C supplements alone did not seem to make a difference, but the combination of vitamins E and C boosted the risk reduction to 53%. Long-term use of vitamin E granted an even stronger risk reduction of 63%. By their nature, though, observational studies cannot fully control for lifestyle factors, so it is possible that people taking vitamin E might also eat better and exercise more, which would influence the results.

So where does all this leave us? Experts uncomfortable with abandoning vitamin E have wondered whether it could be that vitamin E supplements exert a benefit in people who do not already have heart disease or are at low risk for it. Or, perhaps it takes vitamin E longer to exert a clinical benefit than the follow-up period of the studies. Realistically, though, there is no real evidence that this is true.

It might be that we just can't expect vitamin E—or perhaps any other single nutrient—to carry the full burden alone. The antioxidants are a package deal in nature. This group of nutrients, including vitamins E, A, C, selenium, and others, may work best as a team in nature's finely tuned botanical orchestra. The fact that lone vitamin E supplementation appears not to be the magic bullet we had hoped for hints that it might be better to take a balanced, comprehensive array of nutrients rather than depending on high doses of a few key nutrients to carry the load. We will be eagerly awaiting the outcome of ongoing trials of vitamin E combined with other antioxidants.

In addition, vitamin E itself is present in several forms in food, and some researchers believe that this mixture may work best and that perhaps taking too much of one form of vitamin E may blunt the effect of the others.[56]

Preeclampsia Prevention

Preeclampsia is a dangerous complication of pregnancy that involves high blood pressure, swelling of the whole body, and improper kidney function. A double-blind placebo-controlled study of 283 women at increased risk for preeclampsia found that supplementation with vitamin E (400 IU daily) and vitamin C (1,000 mg daily) significantly reduced the chances for developing this disease.[57]

While this research is promising, larger studies are necessary to confirm whether vitamins E and C will actually work. The authors of this study point out that studies of similar size found benefits with other treatments, such as aspirin, that later proved to be ineffective when large-scale studies were performed. Furthermore, keep in mind that we don't know whether such high dosages of these vitamins are absolutely safe for pregnant women.

Tardive Dyskinesia

Tardive dyskinesia consists of involuntary movements of the face, arms, and head, usually caused by the long-term use of antipsychotic drugs. In a double-blind study, 40 subjects were given either placebo or 1,600 IU of vitamin E per day for a period of up to 36 weeks.[58] The vitamin E group did significantly better than those taking placebo. Good results have been seen in smaller, shorter-term studies,[59,60,61] although there have been negative studies too.[62,63] According to one study, 1,600 IU of vitamin E daily is much more effective than 600 IU.[64] However, physician supervision is necessary when using this much.

Immunity

A recent double-blind study suggests that vitamin E may be able to strengthen immunity. In this study, 88 people over the age of 65 were given either placebo or vitamin E at 60 IU, 200 IU, or 800 IU daily.[65] The researchers then gave all participants immunizations against hepatitis B, tetanus, diphtheria, and pneumonia, and looked at subjects' immune response to these vaccinations. The researchers also used a skin test that evaluates the overall strength of the immune response.

The results were impressive. Vitamin E at all dosages significantly increased the strength of the immune response. However, a daily dosage of 200 IU produced the most marked benefits.

Alzheimer's Disease

Preliminary evidence suggests that high-dose vitamin E may slow the progression of Alzheimer's disease.[66] In a double-blind placebo-controlled study, 341 subjects received either 2,000 IU daily of vitamin E, the antioxidant drug selegiline, or placebo. Those given vitamin E took nearly 200 days longer to reach a severe state of the disease than the placebo group. (Selegiline was even more effective.)

Warning: Such high dosages of vitamin E should not be taken except under a doctor's supervision (see Safety Issues).

Low Sperm Count/Infertility

In a double-blind placebo-controlled study of 110 men whose sperm showed subnormal activity, treatment with 100 IU of vitamin E daily resulted in improved sperm activity and higher actual fertility (measured in pregnancies).[67] However, a smaller double-blind trial found no benefit.[68]

Safety Issues

Vitamin E is generally regarded as safe when taken at the recommended dosage of 400 to 800 IU daily. However, vitamin E does have a "blood-thinning" effect that could lead to problems in certain situations. In one study, vitamin E supplementation at the low dose of about 50 IU per day was associated with an increase in hemorrhagic stroke, the kind of stroke caused by bleeding.[69]

Based on its blood-thinning effects, there are concerns that vitamin E could cause problems if it is combined with medications that also thin the blood, such as Coumadin (warfarin), heparin, and aspirin. Theoretically, the net result could be to thin the blood too much, causing bleeding problems. A study that evaluated vitamin E plus aspirin did in fact find an additive effect.[70] In contrast, the results of a study on vitamin E and Coumadin found no evidence of interaction, but it would still not be advisable to combine these treatments except under a physician's supervision.[71]

There is also at least a remote possibility that vitamin E could also interact with herbs that possess a mild blood-thinning effect, such as garlic and ginkgo. Individuals with bleeding disorders such as hemophilia, and those about to undergo surgery or labor and delivery should also approach vitamin E with caution.

⚠ Interactions You Should Know About

If you are taking

- **Blood-thinning drugs**, such as **Coumadin (warfarin)**, **heparin**, or **aspirin:** Seek medical advice before taking vitamin E.
- **Amiodarone:** Vitamin E may help protect you from lung-related side effects.
- High doses of **vitamin E:** Despite some reports, extra vitamin K should not be necessary.[72,73]

VITAMIN K

Supplement Forms/Alternate Names
Vitamin K$_1$ (Phylloquinone), Vitamin K$_2$ (Menaquinone), Vitamin K$_3$ (Menadione)

Principal Proposed Uses
Treating Medication-Induced Vitamin K Deficiency

Other Proposed Uses
Osteoporosis, Menorrhagia (Heavy Menstruation), Nausea

There's a good chance you haven't even heard of vitamin K. However, this obscure member of the vitamin clan is very important for good health. Without it, your blood wouldn't clot properly. There are three forms of vitamin K: K$_1$ (phylloquinone), found in plants; K$_2$ (menaquinone), produced by bacteria in your intestines; and K$_3$ (menadione), a synthetic form.

Vitamin K is used to reverse the effects of "blood-thinning" drugs such as Coumadin (warfarin). Its other proposed uses have little to no supporting evidence as yet.

Requirements/Sources

Vitamin K is an essential nutrient, but you need only a tiny amount of it. The U.S. Recommended Dietary Allowance is

1 mcg per kilogram body weight. This translates into the following

- Infants under 6 months, 5 mcg
    6 to 12 months, 10 mcg
- Children 1 to 3 years, 15 mcg
    4 to 6 years, 20 mcg
    7 to 10 years, 30 mcg
- Males 11 to 14 years, 45 mcg
    15 to 18 years, 65 mcg
    19 to 24 years, 70 mcg
    25 years and older, 80 mcg
- Females 11 to 14 years, 45 mcg
    15 to 18 years, 55 mcg
    19 to 24 years, 60 mcg
    25 years and older, 65 mcg
- Pregnant women, 65 mcg, preferably the K_1 variety (phylloquinone)
- Nursing women, 65 mcg, preferably the K_1 variety

However, a recent study suggests that a higher intake of vitamin K, in the range of 110 mcg daily, might be helpful for preventing osteoporosis.[1]

Vitamin K (in the form of K_1) is found in green leafy vegetables. Kale, green tea, and turnip greens are the best food sources, providing about 10 times the daily adult requirement in a single serving. Spinach, broccoli, lettuce, and cabbage are very rich sources as well, and you can get perfectly respectable amounts of vitamin K in such common foods as oats, green peas, whole wheat, and green beans, as well as watercress and asparagus.

Vitamin K (in the form of K_2) is also manufactured by bacteria in the intestines, and is a major source of vitamin K. Long-term use of antibiotics can cause a vitamin K deficiency by killing these bacteria. Pregnant women, newborn babies, and postmenopausal women are also sometimes deficient in this vitamin.[2,3,4]

Certain drugs can interfere with the action or absorption of vitamin K, including phenytoin (for seizures) and cholestyramine (for high cholesterol).[5,6] The blood-thinning drug Coumadin (warfarin) works by antagonizing the effects of vitamin K. Conversely, vitamin K supplements or intake of foods containing high levels of vitamin K blocks the action of this medication and can be used as an antidote.[7]

People with disorders of the digestive tract, such as chronic diarrhea, celiac sprue, ulcerative colitis, or Crohn's disease, may become deficient in vitamin K.[8–11] Alcoholism can also lead to vitamin K deficiency.[12]

Therapeutic Dosages

For some purposes, vitamin K has been recommended at a daily dose of 150 to 500 mcg. Although such dosages are much higher than required for nutritional purposes, they are not out of the range of what can be reached through eating plenty of green leafy vegetables.

Therapeutic Uses

There are no well-established therapeutic uses of vitamin K, other than its conventional use as an antidote for blood-thinning medications. However, vitamin K may be helpful when you are taking medications that can deplete your body's stores of vitamin K (see Interactions You Should Know About).

Recent evidence suggests that vitamin K supplements can be helpful for preventing osteoporosis.[13 22]

Based on its ability to help blood clot normally, vitamin K has been proposed as a treatment for excessive menstrual bleeding.[23] However, the last actual study testing this idea was carried out more than 55 years ago.[24] Vitamin K has also been recommended for nausea, although there is as yet little evidence that it really works.

What Is the Scientific Evidence for Vitamin K?

Osteoporosis
Vitamin K plays a known biochemical role in the formation of new bone. This has led researchers to look for relationships between vitamin K intake and osteoporosis.

Research has found that people with osteoporosis have much lower blood levels of vitamin K than other people. For example, in a study of 71 postmenopausal women, participants with reduced bone mineral density showed lower serum vitamin K_1 levels than those with normal bone density.[25] Similar results have been seen in other studies.[26,27,28]

A recent report from 12,700 participants in the Nurse's Health Study found that higher dietary intake of vitamin K is associated with a significantly reduced risk of hip fracture.[29]

Interestingly, the most common source of vitamin K used by individuals in the study was iceberg lettuce, followed by broccoli, spinach, romaine lettuce, brussels sprouts, and dark greens. Women who ate lettuce each day had only 55% the risk of hip fracture as those who ate it only weekly. However, among women taking estrogen, no benefit was seen, probably because estrogen is so much more powerful.

Research also suggests that supplemental vitamin K can reduce the amount of calcium lost in the urine.[30,31,32] This is indirect evidence of a beneficial effect on bone.

Taken together, these findings suggest that vitamin K supplements might help prevent osteoporosis.

Safety Issues

Vitamin K is probably quite safe at the recommended therapeutic dosages, since those quantities are easily obtained from food.

Newborns are commonly given vitamin K_1 injections to prevent bleeding problems. Although some have suggested that this practice may increase the risk of cancer,[33] enormous observational studies have found no such connection (one such trial involved more than a million participants).[34,35]

⚠ Interactions You Should Know About

If you are taking

- **Coumadin (warfarin):** Do not take vitamin K supplements or eat foods high in vitamin K except under the supervision of a physician. (You will need to have your medication dosage adjusted.)

- **Dilantin (phenytoin)**, **phenobarbital**, **bile acid sequestrant drugs** (such as **cholestyramine** and **colestipol**), or long-term **antibiotic therapy**: You may need more vitamin K.

ZINC

Supplement Forms/Alternate Names
Chelated Zinc, Zinc Citrate, Zinc Gluconate, Zinc Picolinate, Zinc Sulfate

Principal Proposed Uses
Colds, General Nutritional Supplementation, Pregnancy Support

Other Proposed Uses
Acne, Sickle-Cell Anemia, Ulcers, Rheumatoid Arthritis, Male Infertility, Macular Degeneration, Attention Deficit Disorder, Bladder Infection, Cataracts, Eczema, Periodontal Disease, Psoriasis, and Many Others

---

Zinc is an important element that is found in every cell in the body. More than 300 enzymes in the body need zinc in order to function properly. Although the amount of zinc we need in our daily diet is tiny, it's very important that we get it. However, the evidence suggests that many of us do not get enough. Mild zinc deficiency seems to be fairly common.

Severe zinc deficiency can cause a major loss of immune function, and mild zinc deficiency might impair immunity slightly. For this reason, making sure to get enough zinc may help keep you from catching colds or other infections. But zinc may be helpful for colds in a completely different way, too, by directly killing viruses in the throat. When used in this way, it is taken in the form of lozenges every 2 hours from the first sign of cold symptoms.

Intriguing evidence suggests that zinc supplements may have other specific benefits as well, including helping stomach ulcers heal, relieving symptoms of rheumatoid arthritis, slightly improving acne symptoms, increasing sperm count, and preventing "sickle-cell crisis" (a serious condition in people with sickle-cell anemia).

Requirements/Sources

The U.S. Recommended Dietary Allowance for zinc is as follows

- Infants under 1 year, 5 mg
- Children 1 to 10 years, 10 mg
- Males 11 years and older, 15 mg
- Females 11 years and older, 12 mg
- Pregnant women, 15 mg
- Nursing women, 16 to 19 mg

However, the average diet in the developed world commonly provides less than two-thirds the recommended amount of zinc.[1,2] One study found that more than one-third of pregnant African American women were deficient in zinc.[3] Thus, it may be a wise idea to increase your intake of zinc on general principles.

Children, adolescents, pregnant women, and the elderly are particularly at risk for zinc deficiency, as are those with alcoholism, sickle-cell anemia, diabetes, and kidney disease. The drug AZT, used for AIDS, may impair zinc absorption;[4] the same is true for soy, manganese, and high intake of copper and iron.[5–9] Contrary to previous reports, neither folate nor calcium are likely to significantly affect zinc absorption.[10–13]

Thiazide diuretics ("water pills") can cause excessive loss of zinc in the urine.[14]

Oysters are by far the best food source of zinc—a single serving will give you *10 times* the recommended daily intake! Seeds and nuts, peas, whole wheat, rye, and oats are not nearly as high in zinc, but you can get about 3 mg per serving of these foods.

Zinc can also be taken as a nutritional supplement, in one of many forms. Zinc citrate, zinc acetate, or zinc picolinate may be the best absorbed, although zinc sulfate is less expensive. When you purchase a supplement, you should be aware of the difference between the milligrams of actual zinc the product contains (so-called "elemental zinc") and the total milligrams of the zinc product. For example, 220 mg of zinc sulfate contains 50 mg of zinc. (The rest of the weight is the sulfate.) All figures given in this chapter refer to the amount of actual zinc to take.

Therapeutic Dosages

For most purposes, zinc should simply be taken at the recommended daily requirements listed previously. For best absorption, zinc supplements should not be taken at the same time as high-fiber foods;[15,16] however, many high-fiber foods provide zinc in themselves.

When taking zinc long term it is advisable to take 1 to 3 mg of copper daily as well, because zinc supplements can cause copper deficiency.[17,18] Zinc may also interfere with magnesium[19] and iron[20] absorption. For treatment of colds, much higher doses of zinc are used, although only for a short period of time. The usual dosage is 13 to 23 mg of zinc as zinc gluconate every 2 hours for a week or two (but no longer). The purpose is not to increase zinc levels in your body, but to kill viruses in the back of your throat. It appears that of the common forms of zinc, only zinc gluconate and zinc acetate have the required antiviral properties.[21,22] Also, some sweeteners and flavorings used in lozenges can block zinc's antiviral action. Dextrose, sucrose, mannitol, and sorbitol appear to be fine, but citric acid and tartaric acid are not. The information on glycine as a flavoring agent is a bit equivocal.

Long-term use of relatively high-dose zinc (90 mg daily or more) has been tried for various conditions such as acne, sickle-cell anemia, and rheumatoid arthritis, but medical supervision is essential because of the risk of toxicity (see Safety Issues).

Therapeutic Uses

Good evidence suggests that if you take zinc lozenges every 2 hours at the beginning of a cold, you will recover much more quickly.[23] This approach involves using high doses of zinc for a short period. Long-term zinc supplementation at nutritional doses, which are much lower than what is used for colds, may also reduce the chance of getting sick, but probably only if you are deficient in zinc to begin with.[24,25]

Pregnant women should make sure to get enough zinc. One large double-blind study in zinc-deficient pregnant women found that a standard zinc supplement could significantly improve the birth weight and head size of their newborn children.[26] However, zinc supplements failed to make any difference in another large double-blind study of pregnant women that did not specifically select zinc-deficient women.[27]

Evidence also suggests that, when taken in fairly high dosages, zinc can reduce symptoms of acne.[28]

Zinc may also help prevent the development of sickle-cell crisis in sickle-cell anemia[29] and speed the healing of stomach ulcers.[30,31]

People with rheumatoid arthritis have been found to have lower-than-average blood levels of zinc. Although this doesn't necessarily mean that zinc supplements will reduce symptoms of rheumatoid arthritis, small studies suggest that they might help slightly.[32,33] However, others have shown no benefit at all.[34–37] It may be that zinc is only helpful for those who are zinc deficient in the first place.[38]

One small uncontrolled study found that zinc supplements increased sperm counts and improved fertility for men with low testosterone levels.[39] But no such effect was seen in men whose testosterone levels were normal to begin with.

Although the evidence that it works is not yet meaningful, zinc is sometimes recommended for the following conditions as well: AIDS,[40] Alzheimer's disease,[41–44] anorexia nervosa,[45–48] attention deficit disorder, benign prostatic hyperplasia,[49–55] bladder infection, cataracts, diabetes,[56,57,58] Down's syndrome,[59,60,61] eczema, impotence,[62] inflammatory bowel disease (ulcerative colitis and Crohn's disease),[63–66] macular degeneration,[67,68] osteoporosis,[69] periodontal disease, prostatitis,[70] psoriasis, tinnitus,[71,72] and wound healing.[73,74,75]

What Is the Scientific Evidence for Zinc?

Colds

Numerous studies have evaluated the effects of zinc lozenges for colds. All but one found that zinc lozenges can significantly improve cold symptoms, as long as the right form of zinc is used (zinc gluconate or acetate).[76,77] For example, in a recent double-blind study, 100 nursing home workers with early cold symptoms received either zinc gluconate lozenges or placebo.[78] They took the lozenges until their cold symptoms abated. Overall, the workers who took zinc had fewer days of coughing (2.2 days, compared to 4 for the placebo group), sore throat (1 day versus 3), nasal drainage (4 days versus 7), and headache (2 days versus 3) than the placebo group.

Good results have been seen in several other double-blind studies,[79] including one that used zinc acetate and enrolled about 100 participants.[80] A few studies found no benefit, but a close review of the evidence showed that these studies used forms of zinc lozenges that did not release virus-killing ions into the throat.[81] There has been only one study using the proper chemical form of zinc that did not find benefits, but a cherry flavoring added to the lozenges in that study might have interfered with ion release.[82]

Besides using zinc as a "virus killer," supplementation at nutritional dosages may also help reduce the frequency of colds by strengthening your overall health.

In a 2-year study of nursing home residents, participants given zinc and selenium developed illnesses much less frequently than those given placebo.[83] Of course, it isn't clear from this study which was more helpful, the zinc or the selenium. However, we do know that chronic zinc deficiency weakens the immune system,[84] and studies performed in developing countries using zinc alone have found benefits. For example, a 6-month, double-blind, placebo-controlled study of 609 preschool children in India found that zinc supplements reduced the rate of respiratory infections by 45%.[85] Nine other studies have also found zinc supplements helpful for preventing illness.[86]

Acne

Studies suggest that people with acne have lower-than-normal levels of zinc in their bodies.[87,88,89] This fact alone does not prove that taking zinc supplements will help acne, but several small double-blind studies involving a total of over 300 people have found generally positive results.

In one of these studies, 54 people were given either placebo or 135 mg of zinc as zinc sulfate daily. Zinc produced slight but measurable benefits.[90] Similar results have been seen in other studies using 90 to 135 mg of zinc daily.[91–95] In some studies, however, no benefits were seen.[96,97]

Two studies have compared zinc against a standard treatment for acne, the antibiotic tetracycline. One found that zinc was as effective as tetracycline,[98] but another found the antibiotic more effective.[99]

Keep in mind that the dosages of zinc used in these studies are rather high, and should be used only under a physician's supervision.

Sickle-Cell Anemia

Zinc may also be helpful in preventing "sickle-cell crisis" in individuals with sickle-cell anemia.[100] A placebo-controlled double-blind study treated 145 sickle-cell subjects with either 220 mg of zinc sulfate 3 times daily or placebo. During 18 months of treatment, the zinc-treated subjects had an average of 2.5 crises, compared to 5.3 for the placebo group. However, zinc didn't seem to reduce the severity of a crisis, as measured by the number of days spent in the hospital for each crisis.

Warning: Sickle-cell anemia is far too serious a condition to self-treat, and the relatively high dosages of zinc used in this study should be taken only under the supervision of a doctor (see Safety Issues).

Macular Degeneration

Macular degeneration is one of the most common causes of vision loss in the elderly. One double-blind study of 151 individuals followed for 1 to 2 years found that zinc supplements helped preserve vision.[101] However, another study of 112 individuals found no benefit.[102]

Safety Issues

Zinc seldom causes any immediate side effects other than occasional stomach upset, usually when it's taken on an empty stomach. Some forms do have an unpleasant metallic taste.

However, long-term use of zinc at dosages of 100 mg or more daily can cause a number of toxic effects, including severe copper deficiency, impaired immunity, heart problems, and anemia.[103,104,105] Unless a physician specifically advises you to take a higher dosage, you should stick to the nutritional dosage range described under Requirements/Sources.

Use of zinc can interfere with the absorption of penicillamine and antibiotics in the tetracycline or fluoroquinolone (Cipro, Floxin) families.[106,107,108]

⚠ Interactions You Should Know About

If you are taking

- Medications that reduce stomach acid such as **Zantac (ranitidine)** or **Prilosec (omeprazole)**; **ACE inhibitors**; **oral contraceptives**; **estrogen-replacement therapy**; **thiazide diuretics**; **copper**; or **iron:** You may need to take extra zinc.
- **Antacids**, **soy**, or antibiotics in the **fluoroquinolone** (e.g., Cipro, Floxin) or **tetracycline** families: It may be advisable to separate your doses of zinc and these substances by at least 2 hours.
- **Zinc supplements:** You should also take extra copper, and perhaps magnesium as well because zinc interferes with their absorption. Zinc interferes with iron absorption, too, but you shouldn't take iron supplements unless you know you are deficient.
- **Penicillamine:** You may need extra zinc; however, zinc interferes with penicillamine's absorption so it may be advisable to take zinc and penicillamine at least 2 hours apart.
- **Amiloride:** Do not take zinc unless advised by a physician.

Looking for References?

Due to the large number of references required in a project of this magnitude, we've placed all our research citations conveniently online at www.TNP.com/references/vitamins/. Just click on the vitamin or supplement for which you would like to see a citation and scroll down to the appropriate reference.

If you would prefer to receive an electronic copy of all the references in this book, please send an email request to websupporthlth@primapub.com.

For a hard copy of the references, please call our customer service center at (800) 632-8676 and we will mail you a copy.

Index

About the Series Editors

Steven Bratman, M.D., is Medical Director of TNP.com, as well as Senior Editor for THE NATURAL PHARMACIST™ series of books and all online content. Dr. Bratman is both a strong proponent and vocal critic of alternative treatment, and he believes that alternative medicine has both strengths and weaknesses, just like conventional medicine. This even-handed critique has made him a trusted party on both sides of the debate.

His books include *The Alternative Medicine Sourcebook: A Realistic Evaluation of Alternative Healing Methods* (1997), *The Alternative Medicine Ratings Guide: An Expert Panel Ranks the Best Alternative Treatments for Over 80 Conditions* (Prima Health, 1998), the professional text *Clinical Evaluation of Medicinal Herbs and Other Therapeutic Natural Products* (Prima Health, 1999), and the following titles in THE NATURAL PHARMACIST™ series: *Your Complete Guide to Herbs* (Prima Health, 1999), *Your Complete Guide to Illnesses and Their Natural Remedies* (Prima Health, 1999), *Natural Health Bible, Revised and Expanded 2nd Edition* (Prima Health, 2000), and *Treating Depression* (Prima Health, 1999).

David J. Kroll, Ph.D., is a professor of pharmacology and toxicology at the University of Colorado School of Pharmacy and a consultant for pharmacists, physicians, and alternative practitioners on the indications and cautions for herbal medicine use. He received a degree in toxicology from the Philadelphia College of Pharmacy and Science and obtained his Ph.D. from the University of Florida College of Medicine.

Dr. Kroll has lectured widely and has published articles in a number of medical journals, abstracts, and newsletters. He is also a series editor for THE NATURAL PHARMACIST™ series of books from Prima Health, and is coauthor of both the *Natural Health Bible, Revised and Expanded 2nd Edition* and the professional text *Clinical Evaluation of Medicinal Herbs and Other Therapeutic Natural Products.*

About the Author

Angelo DePalma, Ph.D., was trained as an organic chemist and held the position of senior scientist at a major pharmaceutical company. Dr. DePalma has been reporting on science, technology, and medicine for ten years. He is currently managing editor of Pharmaceutical Online.

Dr. DePalma's contributions to THE NATURAL PHARMACIST series include *Your Complete Guide to Vitamins and Supplements* and co-authorship of *Natural Health Bible*.

Looking for References?

Due to the large number of references required in a project of this magnitude, we've placed all our research citations conveniently online at www.TNP.com/references/vitamins/. Just click on the vitamin or supplement for which you would like to see a citation and scroll down to the appropriate reference.

If you would prefer to receive an electronic copy of all the references in this book, please send an email request to websupporthlth@primapub.com.

For a hard copy of the references, please call our customer service center at (800) 632-8676 and we will mail you a copy.

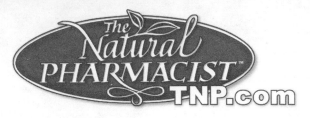

Science-Based Natural Health Information You Can Trust™

TNP.com Is:

- Science-based
- Independent and unbiased
- Up to date
- Balanced—offers both positive and negative findings
- Integrative—includes both conventional and natural treatments
- M.D. and Ph.D. supervised

From Asian Ginseng to Zinc, TNP.com cuts through the hype and tells you what is scientifically proven and what remains unknown about popular natural treatments. Setting a new, high standard of accuracy and objectivity, this Web site takes a realistic look at the herbs and supplements you hear about in the news and provides the balanced information necessary to make informed decisions about your health needs. If you want to be an informed consumer of natural products, TNP.com is the place to start.

Using TNP.com is easy, free, and private. Visit TNP.com now to get science-based natural health information you can trust!

Visit us online at www.TNP.com